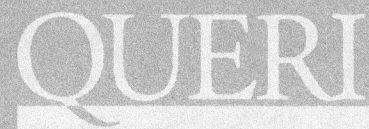

Shared Medical Appointments for Chronic Medical Conditions: A Systematic Review

July 2012

Prepared for:
Department of Veterans Affairs
Veterans Health Administration
Quality Enhancement Research Initiative
Health Services Research & Development Service
Washington, DC 20420

Prepared by:
Evidence-based Synthesis Program (ESP) Center
Durham Veterans Affairs Healthcare System
Durham, NC
John W Williams Jr., M.D., M.H.Sc., Director

Investigators:
Principal Investigator:
David Edelman, M.D.

Co-Investigators:
Jennifer R. McDuffie, Ph.D.
Eugene Oddone, M.D., M.H.Sc.
Jennifer M. Gierisch, Ph.D., M.P.H.
John W. Williams Jr., M.D., M.H.Sc.

Research Associate:
Avishek Nagi, M.S.

Medical Editor:
Liz Wing, M.A.

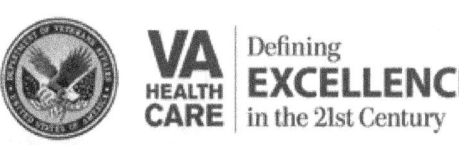

PREFACE

Quality Enhancement Research Initiative's (QUERI's) Evidence-based Synthesis Program (ESP) was established to provide timely and accurate syntheses of targeted healthcare topics of particular importance to Veterans Affairs (VA) managers and policymakers, as they work to improve the health and healthcare of Veterans. The ESP disseminates these reports throughout VA.

QUERI provides funding for four ESP Centers and each Center has an active VA affiliation. The ESP Centers generate evidence syntheses on important clinical practice topics, and these reports help:

- develop clinical policies informed by evidence,
- guide the implementation of effective services to improve patient outcomes and to support VA clinical practice guidelines and performance measures, and
- set the direction for future research to address gaps in clinical knowledge.

In 2009, the ESP Coordinating Center was created to expand the capacity of QUERI Central Office and the four ESP sites by developing and maintaining program processes. In addition, the Center established a Steering Committee comprised of QUERI field-based investigators, VA Patient Care Services, Office of Quality and Performance, and Veterans Integrated Service Networks (VISN) Clinical Management Officers. The Steering Committee provides program oversight, guides strategic planning, coordinates dissemination activities, and develops collaborations with VA leadership to identify new ESP topics of importance to Veterans and the VA healthcare system.

Comments on this evidence report are welcome and can be sent to Nicole Floyd, ESP Coordinating Center Program Manager, at nicole.floyd@va.gov.

Recommended citation: Edelman D, McDuffie JR, Oddone E, Gierisch JM, Nagi A, Williams JW Jr. Shared Medical Appointments for Chronic Medical Conditions: A Systematic Review. VA-ESP Project #09-010; 2012.

This report is based on research conducted by the Evidence-based Synthesis Program (ESP) Center located at the Durham VA Medical Center, Durham, NC, funded by the Department of Veterans Affairs, Veterans Health Administration, Office of Research and Development, Quality Enhancement Research Initiative. The findings and conclusions in this document are those of the author(s) who are responsible for its contents; the findings and conclusions do not necessarily represent the views of the Department of Veterans Affairs or the United States government. Therefore, no statement in this article should be construed as an official position of the Department of Veterans Affairs. No investigators have any affiliations or financial involvement (e.g., employment, consultancies, honoraria, stock ownership or options, expert testimony, grants or patents received or pending, or royalties) that con¬flict with material presented in the report.

TABLE OF CONTENTS

FIGURES

TABLES

EXECUTIVE SUMMARY

BACKGROUND

The most successful health care systems offer ready access to high-quality primary care—an approach that is embedded in the fundamental design of Veterans Affairs (VA) health care and which is consistent with the Institute of Medicine's definition of high-quality care. This definition emphasizes safe, effective, patient-centered, timely, efficient, and equitable health care. Group medical visits are a method to deliver health care that offers the promise of improving these aspects for patients with chronic conditions.

Group visits (or clinics) are a system redesign in which clinicians see multiple patients together in the same clinical setting. Shared medical appointments (SMAs) are a subset of such clinics and are defined by groups of patients meeting over time for comprehensive care for a defining chronic condition or health care state. SMAs usually involve both a person trained or skilled in delivering patient education or facilitating patient interaction and a practitioner with prescribing privileges. SMA sessions typically last 60 to 120 minutes, with time set aside for social integration, interactive education, and medication management, in an effort to achieve improved disease outcomes.

SMAs have been scientifically tested in an array of primary care settings over the last 10 to 15 years. However, there has been great variability among these studies in relation to setting; components included in the intervention; and measurement of clinical, cost, and utilization outcomes. For example, the patient group may stay constant, in an attempt to provide group bonding, or the patients may be allowed to choose sessions from a schedule at their convenience to promote attendance. Like patients, provider teams can be constant or vary over time. This uncertainty regarding the optimal design and impact of SMAs led the VA to commission this evidence synthesis report.

Our objective was to summarize the effects of SMA on staff, patient, and economic outcomes and to evaluate whether the impact varied by clinical condition or specific intervention components.

Key Question 1. For adults with chronic medical conditions, do shared medical appointments (SMAs) compared with usual care improve the following:
- Patient and staff experience?
- Treatment adherence?
- Quality measures such as (a) process of care measures utilized by VA, National Quality Forum, or National Committee for Quality Assurance and (b) biophysical markers (laboratory or physiological markers of health status such as HbA1c and blood pressure)?
- Symptom severity and functional status?
- Utilization of medical resources or health care costs?

Key Question 2. For adults with chronic medical conditions, do the effects of SMAs vary by patient characteristics such as specific chronic medical conditions and severity of disease?

Key Question 3. Is the intensity of the intervention or the components used by SMAs associated with intervention effects?

METHODS

We searched MEDLINE® (via PubMed®), Embase®, CINAHL® , PsycINFO®, and Web of Science for peer-reviewed publications comparing shared medical appointments or group visits with usual care from January 1996 through April 2012. Our search strategy used the National Library of Medicine's medical subject headings (MeSH) keyword nomenclature and text words for group visits, and validated search terms for both randomized controlled trials and relevant observational studies. We limited the search to articles published in the English language involving human subjects 18 years of age and older. We developed our search strategy in consultation with a master librarian. We supplemented the electronic searches with a manual search of citations from a set of key primary articles, review articles and systematic reviews. As a mechanism to assess the risk of publication bias, we searched www.clinicaltrials.gov for completed but unpublished studies.

DATA SYNTHESIS

Using prespecified inclusion and exclusion criteria, we critically analyzed studies to compare their characteristics, methods, findings and quality. When meta-analysis was appropriate, we used random-effects models to synthesize the effects quantitatively, reporting by a weighted difference of the means when the same scale (e.g., blood pressure) was used and a standardized mean difference when the scales (e.g., health-related quality of life) differed across studies. Heterogeneity was examined among the studies using graphical displays and test statistics (Cochran's Q and I^2). We explored heterogeneity in study effects by using subgroup analyses for categorical variables (e.g., study quality) and meta-regression analyses for continuous or discrete variables (e.g., baseline HbA1c, intervention robustness). Our subgroup and meta-regression analyses should be considered hypothesis-generating because they consist of indirect comparisons and thus are subject to confounding. Outcomes not suitable to meta-analyses were described qualitatively

RATING THE BODY OF EVIDENCE

In addition to rating the quality of individual studies, we evaluated the overall strength of evidence (SOE) for each Key Question by assessing the following domains: risk of bias, consistency, directness, precision, strength of association (magnitude of effect), and publication bias. These domains were considered qualitatively, and a summary rating of high, moderate, low, or insufficient SOE was assigned after discussion by two reviewers.

PEER REVIEW

The draft version of the report was reviewed by technical experts and clinical leadership. A transcript of their comments is in an appendix of the full report and elucidates how each comment was considered in the final report.

RESULTS

We identified 1104 unique citations from a combined search of MEDLINE (via PubMed, n=323), CINAHL (n=290), Embase (n=145), PsycINFO (n=157), the Web of Science (n=186) and by manual searching of included study bibliographies and review articles (n=2). After applying eligibility criteria, 25 articles (representing 19 unique studies) were included in the review.

Of the 19 studies, 16 (13 trials) evaluated SMA interventions in patients with diabetes mellitus and 3 (2 trials) evaluated SMAs in older adults with high utilization of medical resources. SMAs were generally led by teams of 1 to 3 clinicians that usually included a physician and/or a registered nurse. Typically, sessions involved fixed patient panels and included individual breakouts for medication management. Group size averaged 6 to 10 members; median visit length was 2 hours and visit frequency ranged from approximately every 3 weeks to every 3 months. Followup ranged from 4 to 48 months. All studies compared SMAs with usual care or enhanced usual care; there were no direct comparisons between SMA and other quality-improvement strategies.

Our search of www.clinicaltrials.gov did not identify any completed but unpublished studies. We found four ongoing studies, three for patients with diabetes and one for those with heart failure.

Key Question 1. For adults with chronic medical conditions, do shared medical appointments (SMAs) compared with usual care improve the following:
- **Patient and staff experience?**
- **Treatment adherence?**
- **Quality measures such as (a) process of care measures utilized by VA, National Quality Forum, or National Committee for Quality Assurance and (b) biophysical markers (laboratory or physiological markers of health status such as HbA1c and blood pressure)?**
- **Symptom severity and functional status?**
- **Utilization of medical resources or health care costs?**

Of the 13 randomized trials that evaluated the effects of SMAs on outcomes for patients with diabetes, ten examined type 2 diabetes only, one examined type 1 only, and two examined a mixed patient population. Other chronic medical conditions were not represented. Studies enrolled patients with poor glucose control (thresholds varied from A1c .6.5% to >9%); a minority required elevated blood pressure or lipids. Only two trials described the effects on patient experience, and neither of those trials showed greater satisfaction among those in SMAs compared with usual care. All studies reported effects on average hemoglobin A1c at the end of the intervention. SMAs were associated with lower A1c than usual care at 4 to 48 months' followup (mean difference=-0.55; 95% CI, -0.99 to -0.11). However, effects varied significantly across studies and this was not explained by study quality. Eight studies reported effects on either total or LDL cholesterol, showing small but statistically nonsignificant treatment effects that varied across studies. Five studies reported effects on systolic blood pressure, showing a consistent and statistically significant effect (mean difference=-5.2; CI, -7.40 to -3.05). Five studies reported large improvements in health-related quality of life (standardized mean difference=-0.84; CI, -1.64 to -0.03), but effects were greater when using a disease-specific measure. Three observational studies examined a more limited set of outcomes, with findings generally consistent with those of the randomized trials.

The effects of SMAs on hospital admissions and emergency department visits were explored in five studies on patients with diabetes. In three of these, admission rates were lower with SMAs, but the result was statistically significant in only one study. Two studies found emergency department visits decreased significantly with SMAs. Four studies reported effects on total costs, but results were mixed. In one, total costs were significantly higher; in another, total costs were significantly lower; in a third, results did not differ significantly; and the fourth was conducted in Europe and so costs may not be applicable to the U.S. health system.

We identified two randomized trials and one observational study that evaluated the effects of SMAs on older adults with high health care service utilization rates. All studies reported positive effects on patient experience with SMAs compared with usual care. Both trials reported effects on overall health status and functional status, but there was no difference compared with usual care for either of these measures. Biophysical outcomes were not reported. All three studies showed fewer hospital admissions in the SMA groups, and both trials reported a statistically significant decrease in emergency department visits with SMAs compared with usual care. Total costs also were lower for the SMA group in each study but varied substantially across studies and did not reach statistical significance for any study.

Table ES-1 summarizes the strength of evidence (SOE) for KQ 1.

Table ES-1. Summary of the strength of evidence for KQ 1

| Population | Number of Studies[a] (Subjects) | Domains Pertaining to SOE | | | | SOE |
		Risk of Bias: Study Design/ Quality	Consistency	Directness	Precision	Effect Estimate (95% CI)
Staff experience						**Insufficient**
Diabetes	0	NA	NA	NA	NA	Not estimable
Older adults	1 (1236)	Obs/Fair	NA	Direct	Imprecise	Not estimable
Patient experience						**Insufficient**
Diabetes	2 (769)	RCT/Fair	Consistent	Direct	Imprecise	No effect
Older adults	2 (444)	RCT/Fair	Inconsistent	Direct	Imprecise	Small to large positive effect
Treatment adherence						**Insufficient**
Diabetes	3 (536)	RCT/Fair	Some inconsistency	Direct	Imprecise	Not estimable
Older adults	0	NA	NA	NA	NA	Not estimable
Biophysical						
Diabetes: A1c	13 (2921)	RCT/Good	Inconsistent	Direct	Some imprecision	MD = -0.55 (-0.99 to -0.11) Moderate SOE

| Population | Number of Studies[a] (Subjects) | Domains Pertaining to SOE | | | | SOE |
		Risk of Bias: Study Design/ Quality	Consistency	Directness	Precision	Effect Estimate (95% CI)
Diabetes: Total Cholesterol	5 (1556)	RCT/Fair	Inconsistent	Direct	Imprecise	MD = -4.9 (-17.8 to 7.9) Low SOE
LDL Cholesterol	5 (997)	RCT/Fair	Inconsistent	Direct	Imprecise	MD -6.6 (-16.1 to 2.8) Low SOE
Diabetes: Blood pressure	5 (1125)	RCT/Good	Consistent	Direct	Some imprecision	MD = -5.2 (-7.4 to -3.1) Moderate SOE
Older adults	0	NA	NA	NA	NA	Not estimable
Health-related quality of life or functional status						
Diabetes	5 (1561)	RCT/Fair	Inconsistent	Direct	Imprecise	SMD = -0.84 (-1.6 to -0.03) Low SOE
Older adults	2 (615)	RCT/Fair	Inconsistent	Direct	Imprecise	Not estimable
Economic						
Diabetes	5 (1339)	RCT/Good	Inconsistent	Direct	Imprecise	*ED visits* lower rates in 2 of 5 studies Insufficient SOE
	5 (1339)	RCT/Good	Consistent	Direct	Some imprecision	*Hospitalizations* lower in 4 of 5 studies Low SOE
	4 (1125)	RCT/Fair	Inconsistent	Direct	Imprecise	*Total costs* range from lower to higher Insufficient SOE
Older adults	2 (615)	RCT/Fair	Consistent	Direct	Imprecise	*ED visits* lower rates in 2 of 2 studies Low SOE
	2 (615)	RCT/Fair	Some inconsistency	Direct	Imprecise	*Hospitalizations* lower in 1 of 2 studies Insufficient SOE
	2 (615)	RCT/Fair	Inconsistent	Direct	Imprecise	*Total costs* lower but not statistically significant Insufficient SOE

[a]Studies (subjects) given are for randomized trials; observational studies were also considered in SOE ratings but are not listed separately in the table.
Abbreviations: CI=confidence interval; ED=emergency department; MD=mean difference; NA=not applicable; RCT=randomized controlled trial; RD=risk difference; RR=risk ratio; SMD=standardized mean difference; SOE=strength of evidence

Key Question 2. For adults with chronic medical conditions, do the effects of SMAs vary by patient characteristics such as specific chronic medical conditions and severity of disease?

No included studies explored the subgroups of patients that would benefit most from an SMA intervention.

Key Question 3. Is the intensity of the intervention or the components used by SMAs associated with intervention effects?

No included studies explored the specific components of an SMA intervention that were most potent. SMA interventions did, however, have certain common components. SMAs were led by teams of 1 to 3 clinicians that included a physician (n=15), clinical pharmacists (n=9; the prescribing clinician in 3 studies), and a registered nurse. The clinical team was multidisciplinary in most studies; pharmacists and licensed mental health professionals participated in almost half the studies. Sessions were designed for closed panels of patients in all but three studies, which used drop-in models. Group size was 6 to 10 members for most studies, with size ranging between 10 and 20 members in 4 studies and as large as 25 members in 1 study. The planned visit frequency ranged from monthly to approximately every 3 months. SMA visits were a median of 2 hours (range 1 to 3.5 hours). At least 16 of 19 studies offered individual breakouts with a physician or clinical pharmacist as part of the SMA design specified that medication changes could be made at group visits. Details of the SMA interventions are given in an appendix of the full report.

We devised an intervention robustness score to attempt to address KQ 3 quantitatively, but it was not associated with treatment effects. More than 70 percent of all studies were similar on six of the seven variables used in the robustness score: (1) whether the team was continuous, (2) whether the group was closed, (3) whether individual breakout sessions were conducted, (4) whether medication changes were made, (5) how long each session was, and (6) whether there was contact outside the session. It is possible that there are other more important variables that are not being measured with current approaches. The strength of evidence for both questions was judged to be insufficient.

RECOMMENDATIONS FOR FUTURE RESEARCH

We used a structured framework to identify gaps in evidence and classify why these gaps exist (Table ES-2).

Table ES-2. Evidence gaps and future research

Evidence Gap	Reason	Type of Studies to Consider
Patients		
Absence of data for patients with conditions other than diabetes mellitus and high utilization	Insufficient information	Single and multisite RCTs Quasi-experimental studies
Interventions		
Uncertain which elements of an SMA intervention are most effective and efficient	Insufficient information	RCTs of head-to-head comparisons of different types of SMAs; Disaggregation trials

Evidence Gap	Reason	Type of Studies to Consider
Outcomes		
Uncertain effects on patient and staff satisfaction	Insufficient information	Nonrandomized or cluster randomized, multisite implementation studies, qualitative studies
Uncertain effects on physiological variables other than HbA1c	Insufficient information	Large scale RCTs Nonrandomized, cluster controlled trials, controlled before-and-after studies, interrupted time series
Uncertain effects on health system costs with the exception of the elderly high utilizers of the health system	Insufficient information	Costs analyses
Uncertain whether there would be unintended consequences to other aspects of the health care system if SMAs were implemented	Insufficient information	Multisite observational studies

Abbreviation: RCT=randomized controlled trial; SMA=shared medical appointment

CONCLUSION

Our review shows that SMAs—typically using closed groups with individual breakouts and opportunity for medication management—improve intermediate clinical outcomes for type 2 diabetes. A smaller literature shows positive effects on patient experience in older adults and the possibility of lower health care utilization. SMAs may be most effective for illnesses such as diabetes that have a phase in which the risk of complication is relatively high while the disease is simultaneously asymptomatic, and in which medication titration and self-management are important. Until further studies are done that allow for comparisons across conditions, the targeting of SMA interventions for chronic conditions other than diabetes will remain speculative.

ABBREVIATIONS TABLE

CI	confidence interval
ED	emergency department
KQ	key question
MD	mean difference
MeSH	medical subject headings
NA	not applicable
NR	not reported
RCT	randomized controlled trial
RD	risk difference
RR	risk ratio
SMA	shared medical appointment
SMD	standardized mean difference
SOE	strength of evidence
VA	Department of Veterans Affairs

EVIDENCE REPORT

INTRODUCTION

Optimal care of chronic illness requires both high-quality care (i.e., excellent clinical outcomes) and ready access to care. However, health care systems struggle with providing access and quality simultaneously—and to achieve both these objectives while simultaneously maintaining staff job satisfaction is a formidable undertaking. Although Veterans Affairs (VA) has made large strides in delivering quality care over the past two decades, quality gaps remain, both gaps in technical quality (e.g., still only 70 to 75% of patients have appropriate blood pressure control[1]) and gaps in timeliness of services. Group medical visits offer the promise of improving the effectiveness, timeliness, and efficiency of health care. Additionally, because clinicians may prefer to work in collaborative, multidisciplinary settings, group medical visits also have the potential to improve staff satisfaction.[2-8]

Group medical visits are defined as multiple patients seen together while in the same clinical setting. A subset of group clinics—referred to as shared medical appointments (SMAs)—is defined by groups of patients meeting over time for comprehensive care, usually involving a practitioner with prescribing privileges, for a defining chronic condition or health care state. SMAs often use educational and/or self-management enhancement strategies, paired with medication management, in an effort to achieve improved disease outcomes.

SMAs have been scientifically studied in an array of primary care settings over the last 10 to 15 years.[3,5,8,13-23] However, there has been great variability among these studies. In particular, the settings of these studies have been heterogeneous; different chronic health care states have been assessed; and the impact on clinical, cost, and utilization outcomes has been variable. Most important, there has been significant variation in the SMA intervention itself—in particular, which types of clinical, educational, and self-efficacy approaches are included in the specific SMA under evaluation. This uncertainty regarding the optimal design and impact of SMAs led the VA to commission this evidence synthesis report.

BACKGROUND

The SMA approach developed as a care redesign strategy over the last 15 years. SMAs are defined as providing group-based, longitudinal medical care for a number of patients who have a common characteristic such as type 2 diabetes.[3,5,8,13-20,22,23] This commonality may be a disease (e.g., diabetes), a demographic (e.g., patients over 65 years of age), or some other health care–related element (e.g., high utilization of services). The patient group may stay constant, in an attempt to provide group bonding, or patients may be allowed to attend sessions chosen from a schedule at their own convenience to promote attendance.

In general, SMAs will have more than one health care provider involved; often the care team will include a person trained or skilled in delivering patient education or facilitating patient interaction (nurse, psychologist) and a prescribing provider empowered to make and initiate a comprehensive care plan. Like patients, providers can either be constant with the same patients or vary over time.

SMA sessions usually last from 60 to 120 minutes. Sessions usually have part of their time set aside for social integration, part set aside for interactive education, and part committed to changes in the care plan for the common condition. The education piece is designed to improve self-management skills; educators will often be formally trained in skills such as motivational interviewing to help patients enhance their self-management. Because they involve both self-management improvement along with medication intensification, SMAs have the potential to coordinate these strategies to maximize the effects of each.

SMAs have been touted as a way to improve key elements of health care, particularly access, outcomes, and cost. Improved access is thought to occur because in a drop-in group structure, patients get their chronic illness care when they want it and/or because a group visit is usually shorter than the amount of time it takes to see all patients in the group one-on-one, thereby improving the provider's throughput and patients' access to that provider. Improved outcomes are thought to occur because (1) the group provides enhanced self-management education due to more time spent in that education, the use of motivational interviewing by the trained facilitator, or the peer support of members of the group, (2) the group provides a focused environment for care of the common condition or unifying characteristic (e.g., older age) without the distractions of multiple other issues that come up in a brief primary care visit, and/or (3) the group provides access to medication changes performed by a provider with special expertise in the common condition or by a team of providers with synergistic knowledge, thus leading the group to function like a specialty referral. Costs are thought to be lowered because the aforementioned efficiency in throughput leads to lower total costs of care or access to a group keeps patients from using acute-care settings for management of chronic illness, saving the costs associated with unnecessary emergency department visits or hospitalizations.

Early studies of SMAs focused on common demographic characteristics (elderly, high utilization) rather than common illnesses.[9,12] However, most recent studies have focused on a common chronic illness as the unifying theme for the SMA, with diabetes the most commonly studied. This may make clinical sense, given that patients with the same chronic illness require self-efficacy for the same self-management skills (e.g., patients with diabetes need to feel empowered to correctly monitor and record blood sugar readings). The disease focus may also be because of the ease of identifying disease-specific clinical outcomes for research studies.

OBJECTIVE OF THIS REPORT

Our objective in this evidence synthesis was to summarize the results of the diverse studies of SMAs in an effort to understand their impact on staff satisfaction, patient experience, and clinical outcomes along with effects on health care utilization. A second objective was to determine whether the impact of SMA visits varies by clinical condition or specific components of the intervention.

METHODS

TOPIC DEVELOPMENT

This review was commissioned by the VA Evidence-based Synthesis Program. The topic was nominated after a topic refinement process that included a preliminary review of published peer-reviewed literature, consultation with internal partners and investigators, and consultation with key stakeholders. We further developed and refined the key questions based on a preliminary review of published peer-reviewed literature in consultation with VA experts.

The final key questions were:

Key Question 1. For adults with chronic medical conditions, do shared medical appointments (SMAs) compared with usual care improve the following:
- Patient and staff experience?
- Treatment adherence?
- Quality measures such as (a) process of care measures utilized by VA, National Quality Forum, or National Committee for Quality Assurance and (b) biophysical markers (laboratory or physiological markers of health status such as HbA1c and blood pressure)?
- Symptom severity and functional status?
- Utilization of medical resources or health care costs?

Key Question 2. For adults with chronic medical conditions, do the effects of SMAs vary by patient characteristics such as specific chronic medical conditions and severity of disease?

Key Question 3. Is the intensity of the intervention or the components used by SMAs associated with intervention effects?

ANALYTIC FRAMEWORK

We followed a standard protocol for all steps of this review; certain methods map to the PRISMA checklist.[24] Our approach was guided by the analytic framework shown in Figure 1.

Figure 1. Analytic framework for evaluating shared medical appointments

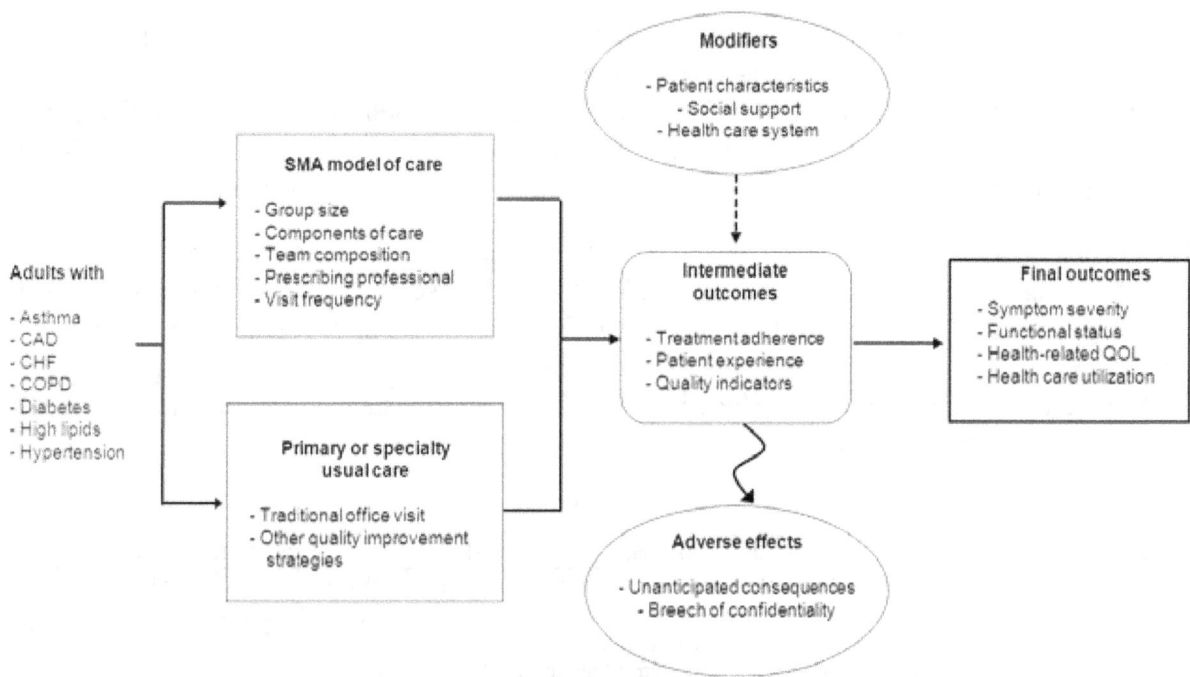

Abbreviations: CAD=coronary artery disease; CHF=congestive heart failure; COPD=chronic obstructive pulmonary disease; KQ=key question; QOL=quality of life; SMA=shared medical appointment

SEARCH STRATEGY

We searched MEDLINE® (via PubMed®), Embase®, CINAHL® , PsycINFO and Web of Science for peer-reviewed publications comparing shared medical appointments or group visits with usual care from January 1996 through September 2011. Our search strategy used the National Library of Medicine's medical subject headings (MeSH) keyword nomenclature and text words for types of visits or clinic appointments, and validated search terms for both randomized controlled trials[25] and relevant observational studies adapted from the Cochrane Effective Practice & Organization of Care Group search version 1.9. Our final search terms included terms for group visits together with terms for trials or relevant observational designs. We limited the search to articles published in the English language involving human subjects 18 years of age and older. The full search strategy is provided in Appendix A. An updated search for publications in PubMed was conducted in April 2012. We developed our search strategy in consultation with an experienced search librarian.

We supplemented the electronic searches with a manual search of citations from a set of key primary articles, three review articles and one systematic review.[3,4,7,10,11,15,18,19,22,26-28] The reference list for identified pivotal articles was manually hand-searched and cross-referenced against our library in order to retrieve additional manuscripts. All citations were imported into two electronic databases: EndNote® Version X5 (Thomson Reuters; Philadelphia, PA) for referencing and DistillerSR (Evidence Partners; Manotick, ON, Canada) for data abstraction. As a mechanism to assess the risk of publication bias, we searched www.clinicaltrials.gov for completed but unpublished studies in March 2012.

STUDY SELECTION

Using prespecified inclusion and exclusion criteria, two reviewers assessed titles and abstracts for relevance to the Key Questions (KQs). Full-text articles identified by either reviewer as potentially relevant were retrieved for further review. Each article retrieved was examined by two reviewers against the eligibility criteria (Table 1). Disagreements on inclusion, exclusion, or major reason for exclusion were resolved by discussion or by a third reviewer.

The criteria to screen articles for inclusion or exclusion at both the title-and-abstract and full-text screening stages are detailed in Table 1. We modified these criteria to include observational studies designs recommended by the Cochrane Effective Practice and Organization of Care Review Group (i.e., controlled before and after, nonrandomized cluster controlled trials, interrupted time-series). Studies excluded at the full-text review stage are listed with the reasons for exclusion in Appendix B.

Table 1. Summary of inclusion and exclusion criteria

Study characteristic	Inclusion criteria	Exclusion criteria
Population	Adults (≥18 years) of age with asthma, coronary artery disease, congestive heart failure, chronic obstructive pulmonary disease, diabetes mellitus, hyperlipidemia, hypertension, or combinations of these chronic medical conditions	Populations selected for individuals with substance abuse disorders
Intervention	"Exposure" must meet all the following criteria: • A series of medical visits (at least two) where at least one health care professional (including a prescribing clinician[a]) cares for a groups of patients • The medical provider addresses each patient's unique medical needs individually, with the potential to make changes in medications, but in the context of the group setting	Study excluded if exposure meets any of the following criteria: • Not a group visit • No prescribing clinician present at the group visit meeting • No plan for adjusting medications when indicated
Comparator	Usual care or other quality improvement strategy	None; study must have a control condition
Outcome	• Patient and/or staff experience • Treatment adherence (attendance, medications, self-management) • Biophysical markers (e.g., HbA1c, blood pressure) • Symptom severity • Functional status • Utilization of medical resources	None
Timing	Outcomes reported at least 3 months from randomization and initiation of intervention	Outcomes reported less than 3 months from randomization and initiation of intervention
Setting	• Outpatient settings; specifically, primary care or specialty clinic/practice • Conducted in North America, Western Europe, Australia/New Zealand	• Conducted in an inpatient or nonmedical community setting (i.e., senior centers, etc.) • Conducted in countries other than those specifically listed as included

Study characteristic	Inclusion criteria	Exclusion criteria
Study design[b]	• Patient or cluster RCTs • Nonrandomized cluster controlled trials • Controlled before-and-after studies • Interrupted time series designs	Cross-sectional studies and other observational study designs not specifically listed as "included" study designs
Publications	• English-language only • Published from 1996 to present • Peer-reviewed article	• Non-English language publication • Published before 1996[c]

[a] A prescribing clinician may be a medical doctor, doctor of osteopathy, advanced practice registered nurse (APRN), physician assistant, or doctor of pharmacy.
[b] Study designs recommended by the Cochrane Effective Practice and Organization of Care Group.
[c] Shared medical appointments were introduced by Beck et al. with their seminal article in 1997.
Abbreviations: HbA1c=glycosylated hemoglobin; KQ=key question; RCT=randomized controlled trial

DATA ABSTRACTION

Before general use, the abstraction form templates designed specifically for this report were pilot-tested on a sample of included articles and revised to ensure that all relevant data elements (Appendix C) were captured and that there was consistency and reproducibility between abstractors. We designed the data abstraction forms for this project to collect the data required to evaluate the specified eligibility criteria for inclusion in this review, as well as population characteristics and other data needed for determining outcomes (e.g., biophysical markers, resource utilization) and risk of bias. We paid particular attention to describing the details of the intervention, including the clinical team (clinical disciplines represented, team size and continuity), characteristics of the patient group (group size, group continuity, inclusion of family members or peer supports), and group visit processes (individual breakouts, medication changes, visit duration, telephone contacts). In addition, we examined the included articles for subgroup analyses of relevance to our key questions.

One investigator abstracted the data, and the second reviewed the completed abstraction form alongside the original article to check for accuracy and completeness. Disagreements were resolved by consensus or by obtaining a third investigator's opinion if consensus could not be reached by the first two. We supplemented abstraction of published data by contacting authors for missing information. We contacted 11 of 19 authors; of these, 7 replied with the requested information.

QUALITY ASSESSMENT

We also abstracted data necessary for assessing quality and applicability, as described in the Agency for Healthcare Research and Quality's (AHRQ's) *Methods Guide for Effectiveness and Comparative Effectiveness Reviews*.[29] For RCTs, these key quality criteria consisted of (1) adequacy of randomization and allocation concealment, (2) comparability of groups at baseline, (3) blinding, (4) completeness of followup and differential loss to followup, (5) whether incomplete data were addressed appropriately, (6) validity of outcome measures, and (7) conflicts of interest (Appendix D). Using these quality criteria, we assigned a summary quality score (good, fair, poor) to individual RCTs studies as defined in the *Methods Guide*.

Threats to internal validity of systematic review conclusions based on observational studies were identified through assessment of the body of observational literature as a whole, with an examination of characteristics of individual studies.[29,30] Study-specific issues that were considered include (1) potential selection bias (i.e., degree of similarity between intervention and control patients), (2) performance bias (i.e., differences in care provided to intervention and control patients not related to the study intervention), (3) attribution and detection bias (i.e., whether outcomes were differentially detected between intervention and control groups), and (4) magnitude of reported intervention effects (see the section on "Selecting Observational Studies for Comparing Medical Interventions" in the *Methods Guide*).[29] For each study, one investigator assigned a summary quality rating for "hard outcomes" (e.g., laboratory measures) and a separate rating for "soft" outcomes (e.g., staff experience), which were then reviewed by a second investigator; disagreements were resolved by consensus or by a third investigator if agreement could not be reached.

DATA SYNTHESIS

We critically analyzed studies to compare their characteristics, methods, and findings. We then determined the feasibility of completing a quantitative synthesis (i.e., meta-analysis) by exploring the volume of relevant literature, the completeness of the results reporting and the conceptual homogeneity of the studies. Because the elderly and individuals with diabetes mellitus are high utilizers of the health care system and are distinct groups of clinical patients with distinct primary endpoints, we examined the groups of studies as they pertained to these target conditions separately.

When a meta-analysis was appropriate, we used random-effects models to synthesize the available evidence quantitatively. For other outcomes we analyzed the results qualitatively. The outcomes amenable to meta-analysis were continuous; we therefore summarized these outcomes by a weighted difference of the means when the same scale (e.g., blood pressure) was used and a standardized mean difference when the scales (e.g., health-related quality of life) differed across studies. We present summary estimates (standardized so that a negative value favors SMA) and 95 percent confidence intervals (95% CIs). **Heterogeneity was examined** among the studies using graphical displays and test statistics (Cochran's Q and I^2); the I^2 describes the percentage of total variation across studies due to heterogeneity rather than to chance.[31] Heterogeneity was categorized as low, moderate, or high based on I^2 values of 25 percent, 50 percent, and 75 percent respectively. We explored heterogeneity in study effects by using subgroup analyses for categorical variables (e.g., study quality) and meta-regression analyses for continuous or discrete variables (e.g., baseline HbA1c, intervention robustness). We constructed a "robustness score" that could range from 0 to 9, based on 7 intervention elements that were chosen a priori: theoretical framework guiding the intervention, individual breakouts, continuity between patients and clinical team, scheduled visits above the median, and medication changes. The latter two characteristics were scored 0 (absent) or 2 (present); all other items were scored as 0 or 1. We conducted a sensitivity analyses by using only studies whose populations had type 2 diabetes. Our subgroup and meta-regression analyses should be considered hypothesis-generating because they consist of indirect comparisons (across studies that may differ in ways other than the target condition) and thus are subject to confounding.

All basic analyses were conducted using Review Manager (RevMan) 5.1.4. (Copenhagen: The Nordic Cochrane Centre, The Cochrane Collaboration, 2011). Meta-regression analyses were conducted using Comprehensive Meta-Analysis software (Version 2; Biostat, Englewood, NJ).

RATING THE BODY OF EVIDENCE

In addition to rating the quality of individual studies, we evaluated the overall quality of the evidence for each KQ as described in the *Methods Guide*.[29] In brief, this approach requires assessment of four domains: risk of bias, consistency, directness, and precision. Additional domains considered were strength of association (magnitude of effect) and publication bias. For risk of bias, we considered basic (e.g., RCT) and detailed study design (e.g., adequate randomization). We used results from meta-analyses when evaluating consistency (forest plots, tests for heterogeneity), precision (confidence intervals), strength of association (weighted mean difference), and publication bias (clinicaltrials.gov survey). Optimal information size and consideration of whether the confidence interval crossed the clinical-decision threshold using a treatment model were also used when evaluating precision.[32] These domains were considered qualitatively, and a summary rating of high, moderate, low, or insufficient strength of evidence was assigned after discussion by two investigators. This four-level rating scale consists of the following definitions:

- High—Further research is very unlikely to change our confidence on the estimate of effect.
- Moderate—Further research is likely to have an important impact on our confidence in the estimate of effect and may change the estimate.
- Low—Further research is very likely to have an important impact on our confidence in the estimate of effect and is likely to change the estimate.
- Insufficient—Evidence on an outcome is absent or too weak, sparse, or inconsistent to estimate an effect.

When a rating of high, moderate, or low was not possible or was imprudent to make, a grade of insufficient was assigned.[33] We also considered the risk of publication bias. Publication bias was addressed through a careful search of www.clinicaltrials.gov for identification of any study completed but unpublished or ongoing. For the single outcome with at least 10 studies, we used graphical (e.g., funnel plots) and test statistics (e.g., Beggs test) to detect publication bias; these methods do not perform well with fewer than 10 studies and thus were not performed for the other outcomes.[34,35]

PEER REVIEW

A draft version of the report was reviewed by technical experts and clinical leadership. A transcript of their comments can be found in Appendix E, which elucidates how each comment was considered in the final report.

RESULTS

LITERATURE FLOW

The flow of articles through the literature search and screening process is illustrated in Figure 2. We identified 1101 unique citations from a combined search of MEDLINE (via PubMed, n=323), CINAHL (n=290), Embase (n=145), PsycINFO (n=157) and the Web of Science (n=186). Manual searching of included study bibliographies and review articles identified 2 additional citations for a total of 1104 citations. After applying inclusion/exclusion criteria at the title-and-abstract level, 95 full-text articles were retrieved and screened. Of these, 70 were excluded at the full-text screening stage, leaving 25 articles (representing 19 unique studies) for data abstraction. All studies compared shared medical appointments with usual care or enhanced usual care; there were no direct comparisons between types of quality-improvement strategies. Our search of www.clinicaltrials.gov did not suggest publication bias. There were no completed studies that were unpublished. We found four ongoing studies (Appendix F), one of which had a methods paper. Interestingly, in light of the narrowness of the medical conditions in which SMA has been tested, one study is on patients with heart failure.

Figure 2. Literature flow diagram for randomized controlled trials and observational studies on SMA

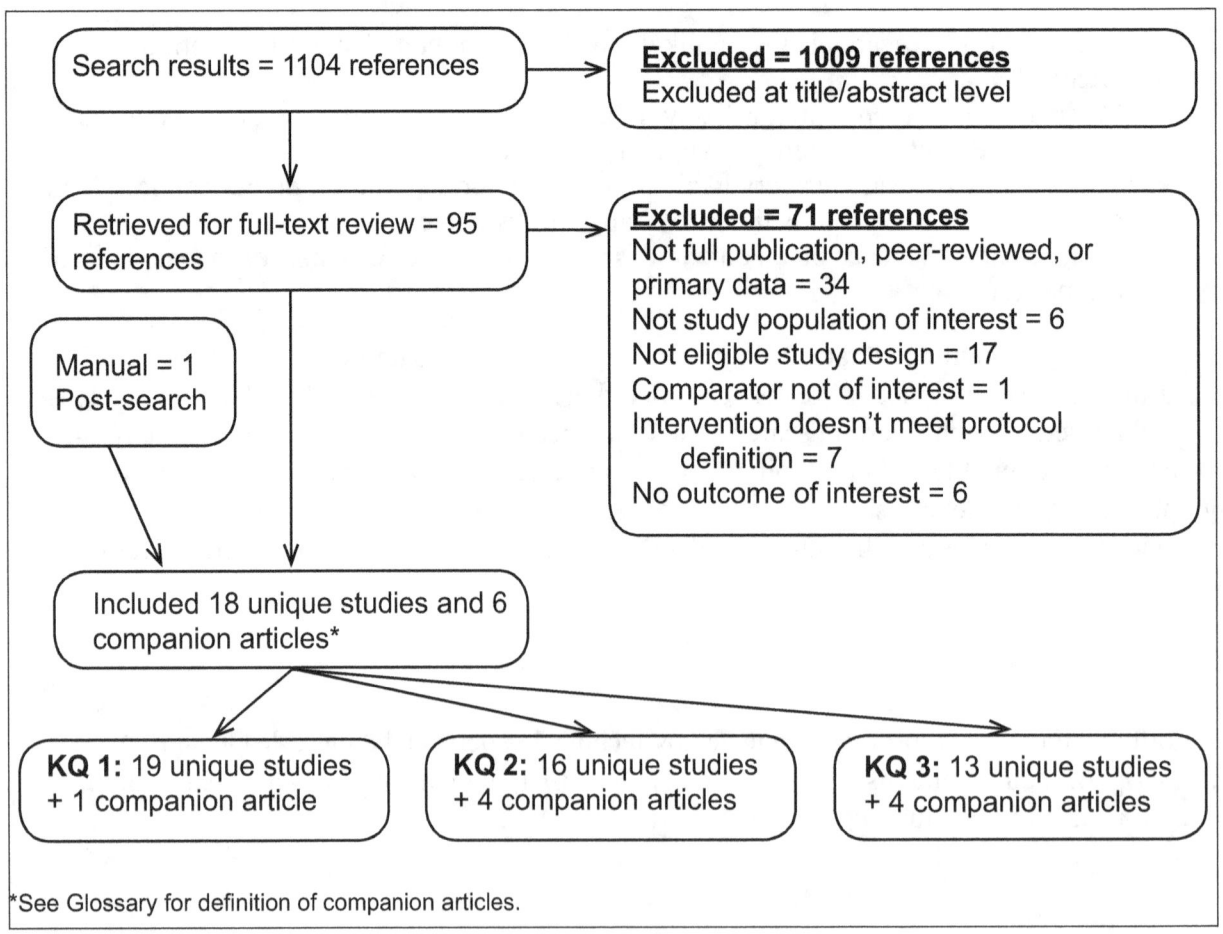

*See Glossary for definition of companion articles.

Abbreviations: KQ=key question; SMA=shared medical appointment

STUDY CHARACTERISTICS

Of the 19 studies, 16 (13 trials) evaluated SMA interventions in patients with diabetes mellitus and 3 (2 trials) evaluated SMAs in older adults with high utilization of medical resources. Most studies were conducted in primary care settings that are part of integrated health systems in the United States (Table 2). Of the 19 studies, 15 reported outcomes at 1 year or later. Detailed study characteristics are given in Appendix G.

Table 2. Overview of studies evaluating SMA

Study Characteristic	Adults With Diabetes	Older Adults
N studies (participants)	16 (3221)[a]	3 (1851)
Mean age of sample: median (range)	60.8 (27 to 69.8)	74.1 (73.5 to 78.2)
Setting: N studies (participants)		
Primary care	13 (2232)	3 (1851)
Medical Subspecialty	3 (989)	0
Health care system: N studies (participants)		
Government (VA, FQC)	7 (771)	0
Private integrated system (HMO)	2 (892)	3 (1851)
University-affiliated clinic	7 (1558)	0
Country: N studies (participants)		
United States	13 (2232)	3 (1851)
Europe	3 (989)	0
Study design: N studies (participants)		
Randomized controlled trial	13 (2921)	2 (615)
Observational	3 (300)	1 (1236)
Sites: N studies (participants)		
Single	14 (2106)	1 (321)
Multisite	2 (1115)	2 (1530)
Study duration[b]: N studies (participants)		
6 to 12 months	4 (410)	0
>12 months	12 (2811)	3 (1851)

[a]Participant number is based on the number randomized.
[b]Study duration is measured from time of randomization to most distal followup.
Abbreviations: FQC=Federally qualified center; VA=Veterans Administration; HMO=health maintenance organization

Characteristics of Shared Medical Appointments

In the studies we assessed, SMAs were led by teams of 1 to 3 clinicians that included a physician (n=15), clinical pharmacists (n=9; the prescribing clinician in 3 studies) and a registered nurse (Table 3). The clinical team was multidisciplinary in most studies; pharmacists and licensed mental health professionals participated in almost half the studies. Sessions were designed for closed panels of patients in all but three studies; these later studies used drop-in models. Group size was 6 to 10 for most studies, with group size ranging between 10 and 20 in 4 studies and group size as large as 25 members in one study. The planned visit frequency ranged from approximately every 3 weeks to every 3 months. SMA visits were a median of 2 hours (range 1 to 3.5 hours).

At least 16 of 19 studies offered individual breakouts with a physician or clinical pharmacist as part of the SMA design specified that medication changes could be made at group visits. Three studies did not report this information. About half the studies invited participation by family members or friends. Three studies described the educational approach as "patient-centered adult learning,"[20-22] and two studies used the stages-of-change model to design the intervention;[8,26] no other study described a theoretical model. In about half the studies, patients participated in selecting or prioritizing educational topics, and printed materials were tailored to the individual patient. Few studies used telephone contact as a part of the SMA intervention. Details of the SMA interventions are given in Appendix H.

Table 3. Characteristics of shared medical appointment interventions

Characteristic	Diabetes (16 Studies)	Older Adults (3 Studies)
Intervention team disciplines: N studies (participants)		
Medical doctor	12 (2731)	3 (1851)
Nurse practitioner	3 (298)	1 (1236)
Pharmacist	8 (1609)	1 (294)
Registered nurse	10 (2791)	2 (615)
Dietician	4 (1208)	0
Physical therapist/exercise specialist	3 (269)	1 (294)
Psychologist/Behavioral specialist	3 (326)	1 (321)
Health educator	3 (1116)	0
Social worker	2 (164)	0
Other[a]	6 (1238)	2 (1530)
Intervention team size		
Median number of members (range)	2.5 (2 to 7)	2.5 (2 to 3)
Average visit duration		
Median minutes (range)	120 (60 to 210)	120 (90 to 120)
Number of planned visits		
Median (range)	7.5 (4 to 36)	12 (12 to 24)
Medication changes made during sessions		
Yes	13 (2217)	3 (1851)
Not reported/unclear	3 (995)	0
Individual breakouts: N studies (participants)		
Yes	12 (2850)	3 (1851)
No	1 (88)	0
Not reported/unclear	3 (273)	0
Behavioral components		
Licensed mental health professional led group education session		
Yes	6 (1356)	1 (321)
No	9 (1149)	2 (1530)
Not reported/unclear	1 (707)	0
Family/friend participation		
Yes	7 (1346)	2 (615)
No	4 (527)	0
Not reported/unclear	5 (1169)	1 (1236)
Patient-clinician group continuity: N studies (participants)		
Group member continuity[b]		
Closed	13 (2942)	2 (1557)
Open/drop-in	3 (270)	1 (294)
Team continuity		
Consistent care team	12 (2120)	2 (1530)
Care team changes/rotates	3 (989)	1 (321)
Not reported/unclear	1 (103)	0
Some intervention components delivered by telephone		
Yes	2 (424)	1 (312)
No	10 (2385)	1 (294)
Not reported/unclear	4 (403)	1 (1236)

[a]Disciplines that were present on only one team: occupational therapist, medical assistant, research assistant or undefined; there were no physician assistants used, although this would be a valid clinical discipline for teams.
[b]Group membership was classified as closed when the same group of patients were scheduled for each SMA visit.

Comparison Condition

In all studies, the comparison condition was some form of usual care. This care was inconsistently described. Three studies by one group[20-22] and one other study[18] used a structured or enhanced form of usual care. In one study,[22] this care consisted of individual visits with a forced interval of 3 months; in another study,[18] this was VA usual care supplemented with a single diabetes education session; and in the other two studies,[20,21] usual primary care was enhanced by one-on-one education sessions with the group facilitator. Three studies conducted in the VA[8,26,36] described usual care at some length, including average visit frequencies of 4 months, online clinical tools, electronic medical records with clinical reminders related to diabetes care, and a full range of referral services including diabetes education. Three other VA studies[5,14,15] very briefly described usual care. The other nine studies did not describe usual care at all.

KEY QUESTION 1: For adults with chronic medical conditions, do shared medical appointments (SMAs) compared with usual care improve the following:

- **Patient and staff experience?**
- **Treatment adherence?**
- **Quality measures such as (a) process of care measures utilized by VA, National Quality Forum, or National Committee for Quality Assurance and (b) biophysical markers (laboratory or physiological markers of health status such as HbA1c and blood pressure)?**
- **Symptom severity and functional status?**
- **Utilization of medical resources or health care costs?**

Effects of Shared Medical Appointments on Clinical, Process, and Economic Outcomes

The outcomes reported varied widely across studies and between studies for adults with diabetes and older adults. We describe the results separately for these two populations.

Effect of SMAs on Outcomes for Adults With Diabetes

Patient selection for SMA studies among patients with diabetes

Patient characteristics are reported in Table 4. Briefly, 10 of 15 studies required patients to be "out of control" with regard to their A1c; however, this inclusion floor varied from a low of 6.5% to a high of 9.0%. Four studies required elevated blood pressure, and two required elevated lipids. Other criteria were used by no more than two studies (e.g., efforts to assure that diabetes was type 2, insulin-requiring, high utilization in past year).

We identified 13 randomized trials that evaluated the effects of SMAs on outcomes for patients with diabetes.[3,8,14,15,17-22,26,36,37] Of these, ten enrolled only patients with type 2 diabetes,[3,8,14,15,17,18,20,22,26,36] two enrolled mixed samples,[19,37] and one enrolled only patients with type 1 diabetes.[21] Three observational studies evaluated SMAs.[5,13,16] All but one of these 16 studies compared SMAs with usual care. One study[18] compared SMAs with a traditional, two-session, diabetes education intervention. Study quality was rated as good for 6 trials, fair for 6 trials and 2 observational studies, and poor for the two remaining studies. For trials, methodological problems included (1) failure to describe allocation concealment (n=9), (2) outcomes assessed without blinding to intervention (n=6), and (3) an inadequate approach to addressing incomplete data (n=6). Except for the study in patients with type 1 diabetes, patients were older adults with representative gender and racial mixes (Table 4).

Table 4. Study details for SMAs enrolling adults with diabetes

Characteristic	Randomized Trials	Observational studies
N studies (participants)	13 (2921)[a]	3 (300)
Median age of sample (range)[b]	60.8 (29 to 69.8)	59.4 (56.8 to 61.0)
Sex: N (%)		
Male	1585 (54.3%)	93 (31.0%)
Female	1137 (38.9%)	128 (42.7%)
Not reported (3 studies)	190 (6.8%)	79 (26.3%)
Race: N (%)[c]		
African American	425 (16.4%)	–
White	952 (36.7%)	–
Other	127 (4.9%)	–
Not reported	1088 (42.0%)	300 (100%)
Study quality: N (%)		
Good	6 (46%)	0
Fair	6 (46%)	2 (67%)
Poor	1 (8%)	1 (33%)

[a]Participant number is based on the number included in description of population characteristics, which is a smaller sample than those randomized.
[b]Mean age was not reported in one study.
[c]Of studies reporting race, 329 participants were not accounted for; therefore, percentage is of n=2592.

Treatment Experience and Adherence Outcomes

Only two trials[21,37] described the effects on patient experience, and none reported effects on staff experience. Neither of those trials showed greater satisfaction among those in SMAs compared with usual care. One study reported no effects on medication adherence,[3] another reported no effects on blood glucose self-monitoring,[20] and two studies reported mixed effects on self-management behaviors.[19,36] In both studies, patients in the SMA group increased the frequency of home glucose monitoring more than in the usual care group. Foot self-exams increased significantly in one study,[36] and exercise time increased by a statistically nonsignificant degree compared with usual care.

Effects on medication treatment were reported in 8 of 13 studies, but outcomes were reported inconsistently. One of four studies[26] reported more medication starts or dose titrations for oral hypoglycemic medications, and one of two studies[8] reported more insulin starts and increased insulin doses for the SMA group. One of three studies[26] found more antihypertensive medication starts or dose titrations overall in the SMA intervention group, and two studies[8,15] found greater use of dose titrations for selected antihypertensive medications. Only one of five studies[8] found a statistically significant increase in lipid-lowering medications and this was only for niacin. Most of the positive intervention effects were in studies led by clinical pharmacists. Patient or staff experience was not reported in any of the observational studies.

Biophysical Outcomes

Hemoglobin A1c. Figure 3 shows the forest plots for the random-effects meta-analyses of the effect of SMAs on glucose. All studies reported effects on average glucose (A1c) at the end of the intervention, assessed at 6 months to 4 years. SMAs were associated with lower A1c than usual care (mean difference=-0.55; 95% CI, -0.99 to -0.11). However, effects varied significantly across studies (Q=179.9, df=12, p < 0.001; I^2 =93%)—variability that was not explained by study quality. Because of the variability in effects between studies, we conducted analyses to evaluate this variability. First, we conducted a sensitivity analysis, excluding the study in patients with type 1 diabetes,[21] but variability remained high (I^2=94%). Next, we used meta-regression analyses to evaluate the association between baseline A1c and intervention robustness with treatment effects. Neither baseline A1c nor intervention robustness (B=0.02 decrease in A1c per 1 point increase in robustness; CI, -0.23 to 0.26) was associated with treatment effects (p=0.90). Thus, SMAs were associated with a mean decrease in A1c, but effects varied markedly and were not explained by factors we hypothesized a priori to be associated with variation in treatment effect.

Effects of SMAs on glucose from the observational studies were generally consistent with the trial data. Two of the three observational studies[5,13] found statistically significant reductions in A1c from baseline to followup among patients participating in SMAs. Only one study[5] compared this change with a control group, finding a statistically significant benefit from SMA participation (p=0.002).

Figure 3. Effects of shared medical appointments on hemoglobin A1c

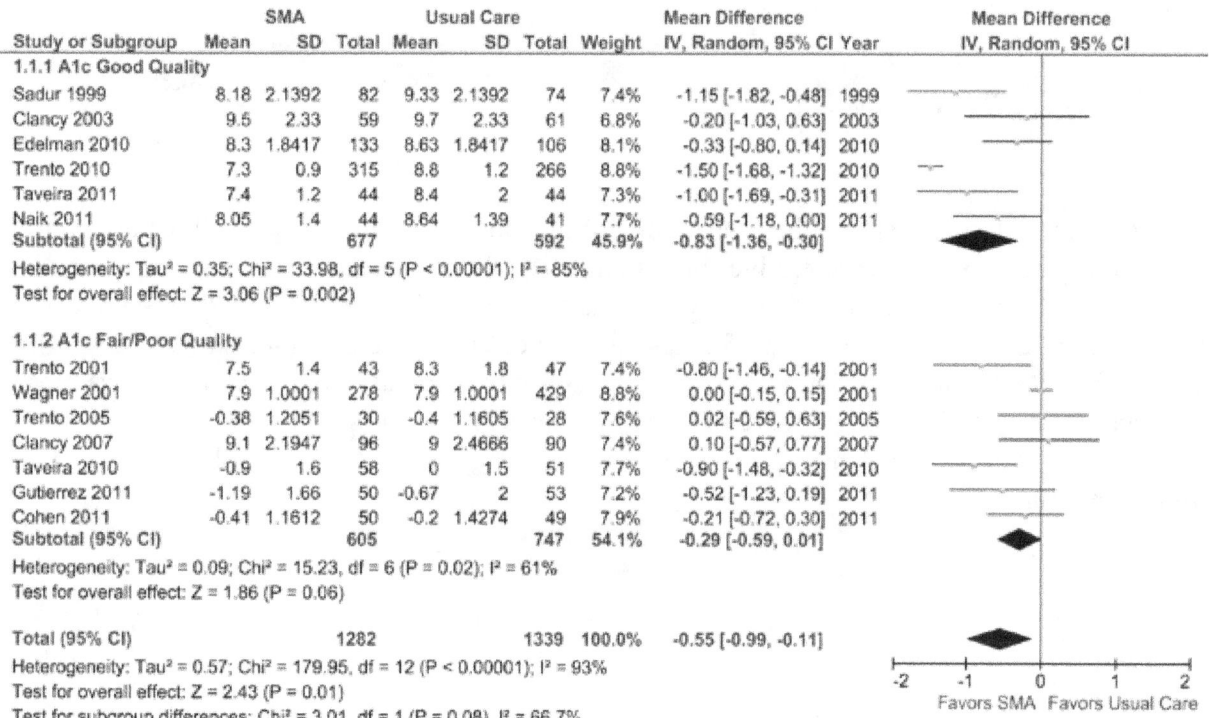

Cholesterol. Figures 4 and 5 show the forest plots for the random-effects analyses of the effect of SMAs on total cholesterol (5 studies) and LDL cholesterol (5 studies). For both outcomes, SMAs were associated with a statistically nonsignificant decrease in cholesterol. For each outcome, treatment effects varied significantly across studies. Because of the small number of studies, we did not complete meta-regression analyses to examine variability in treatment effects. One additional study[17] reported a statistically nonsignificant increase in the proportion of patients achieving an LDL of less than 100—findings that are consistent with the analysis of mean change in LDL. Only two of the observational studies reported effects on cholesterol. Both found reductions in LDL cholesterol, but only one[5] compared the SMA with the control group, and the differences were not statistically significant.

Figure 4. Effects of shared medical appointments on total cholesterol

Study or Subgroup	SMA Mean [mg/dl]	SD [mg/dl]	Total	Usual Care Mean [mg/dl]	SD [mg/dl]	Total	Weight	Mean Difference IV, Random, 95% CI [mg/dl]	Year
Wagner 2001	202.8	42.2	278	204.6	42.2	429	24.5%	-1.80 [-8.17, 4.57]	2001
Trento 2001	220.4	46.4	43	216.6	46.4	47	16.5%	3.80 [-15.39, 22.99]	2001
Clancy 2003	195.6	41.7	59	196.9	41.7	61	19.3%	-1.30 [-16.22, 13.62]	2003
Trento 2005	184.8	37.9	30	179.8	44.9	28	15.1%	5.00 [-16.46, 26.46]	2005
Trento 2010	188.7	37.1	315	211.5	36.4	266	24.6%	-22.80 [-28.79, -16.81]	2010
Total (95% CI)			**725**			**831**	**100.0%**	**-4.92 [-17.82, 7.97]**	

Heterogeneity: Tau² = 166.43; Chi² = 28.93, df = 4 (P < 0.00001); I² = 86%
Test for overall effect: Z = 0.75 (P = 0.45)

Favors SMA Favors Usual Care

Figure 5. Effects of shared medical appointments on LDL cholesterol

Study or Subgroup	Favors SMA Mean [mg/dl]	SD [mg/dl]	Total	Usual Care Mean [mg/dl]	SD [mg/dl]	Total	Weight	Mean Difference IV, Random, 95% CI [mg/dl]	Year
Clancy 2003	107.6	31.2	59	116.2	31.2	61	19.0%	-8.60 [-19.77, 2.57]	2003
Trento 2010	107.9	36.4	315	127.9	37.5	266	23.3%	-20.00 [-26.04, -13.96]	2010
Taveira 2010	82.8	24.1	58	85.2	26.7	51	20.4%	-2.40 [-12.00, 7.20]	2010
Taveira 2011	92.5	24.3	44	93.9	30.6	44	18.6%	-1.40 [-12.95, 10.15]	2011
Cohen 2011 (1)	-9.4	23.716	50	-11.53	33.2134	49	18.8%	2.13 [-9.26, 13.52]	2011
Total (95% CI)			**526**			**471**	**100.0%**	**-6.64 [-16.11, 2.82]**	

Heterogeneity: Tau² = 90.57; Chi² = 19.46, df = 4 (P = 0.0006); I² = 79%
Test for overall effect: Z = 1.38 (P = 0.17)

Favors SMA Favors Usual Care

(1) Mean change

Blood pressure. Figure 6 shows the forest plots for the random-effects analyses of the effect of SMAs on systolic blood pressure. Five studies reported effects on systolic blood pressure;[3,8,22,26,36] four of these were conducted in VA. SMAs were associated with improved blood pressure control (MD, -5.22; 95% CI, -7.40 to -3.05). Results were consistent across studies (Q=1.82, df=4, p=0.77, I²=0%). Of the three observational studies, only one[5] found a statistically significant pre–post change in systolic blood pressure for the SMA participants. In this study, the blood pressure effects were also greater for the SMA group (-14.93 mmHg) than for the control group (-2.54 mmHg, p=0.04).

Figure 6. Effects of shared medical appointments on systolic blood pressure

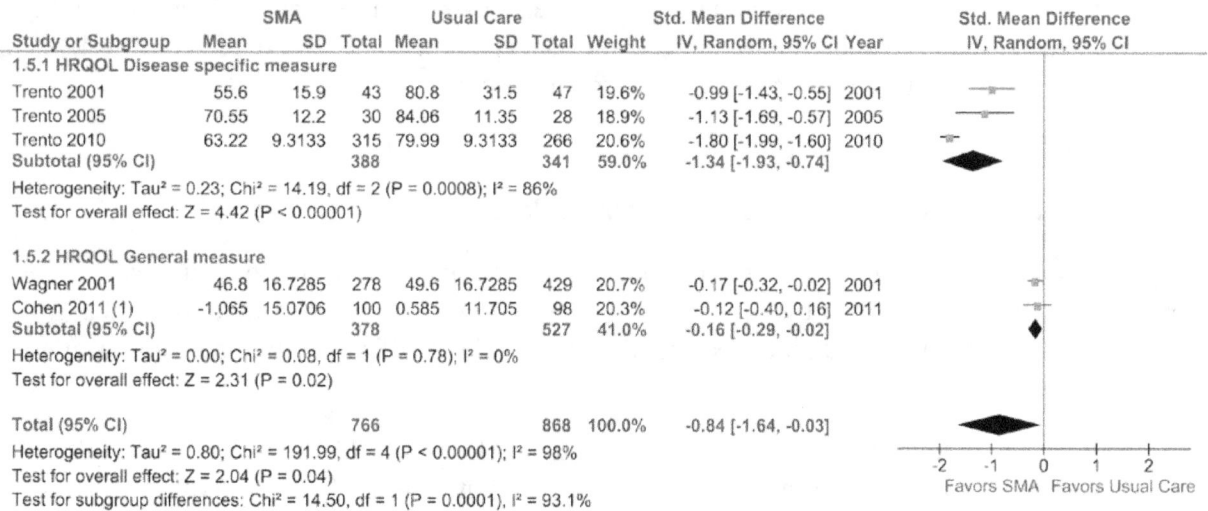

Study or Subgroup	SMA Mean [mmHg]	SD [mmHg]	Total	Usual Care Mean [mmHg]	SD [mmHg]	Total	Weight	Mean Difference IV, Random, 95% CI [mmHg]
Edelman 2010	139.2	21.5523	133	146.5	21.5523	106	15.6%	-7.30 [-12.80, -1.80]
Taveira 2010	-7.3	20.3	58	-1.7	19.6	51	8.4%	-5.60 [-13.10, 1.90]
Trento 2010	138.01	16.1	295	142.43	18.9929	266	55.1%	-4.42 [-7.35, -1.49]
Cohen 2011 (1)	-9.19	20.2676	50	-0.8	16.746	49	8.8%	-8.39 [-15.71, -1.07]
Taveira 2011	123.4	12.3	44	127	17.3	44	12.0%	-3.60 [-9.87, 2.67]
Total (95% CI)			580			516	100.0%	-5.22 [-7.40, -3.05]

Heterogeneity: Tau² = 0.00; Chi² = 1.82, df = 4 (P = 0.77); I² = 0%
Test for overall effect: Z = 4.71 (P < 0.00001)

(1) Cohen 2011 and Traveira 2010 is mean change

Health-Related Quality-of-Life Outcomes

Figure 7 shows the random-effects meta-analysis of the effect of SMAs on health-related quality of life (HRQOL). Six studies[17,20-22,36,37] reported measuring HRQOL, but only five of these reported outcomes.[20-22,36,37] The studies by Trento et al. measured HRQOL with the Diabetes Quality-of-Life Measure, Cohen et al. reported the mental and physical components of the SF-36, and Wagner et al. reported the general health subscale of the SF-36. Because these measures differ, we analyzed the data using standardized mean difference. SMAs were associated with a large improvement in HRQOL (SMD -0.84; 95% CI, -1.64 to -0.03), but effects varied substantially across studies (Q=191.99, df=4, p<0.001; I²=98%). There were too few studies to evaluate the variability in treatment effects quantitatively. However, the studies with the smallest effects[36,37] used general rather than disease-specific measures.

Figure 7. Effects of shared medical appointments on health-related quality of life

Study or Subgroup	SMA Mean	SD	Total	Usual Care Mean	SD	Total	Weight	Std. Mean Difference IV, Random, 95% CI	Year
1.5.1 HRQOL Disease specific measure									
Trento 2001	55.6	15.9	43	80.8	31.5	47	19.6%	-0.99 [-1.43, -0.55]	2001
Trento 2005	70.55	12.2	30	84.06	11.35	28	18.9%	-1.13 [-1.69, -0.57]	2005
Trento 2010	63.22	9.3133	315	79.99	9.3133	266	20.6%	-1.80 [-1.99, -1.60]	2010
Subtotal (95% CI)			388			341	59.0%	-1.34 [-1.93, -0.74]	

Heterogeneity: Tau² = 0.23; Chi² = 14.19, df = 2 (P = 0.0008); I² = 86%
Test for overall effect: Z = 4.42 (P < 0.00001)

1.5.2 HRQOL General measure									
Wagner 2001	46.8	16.7285	278	49.6	16.7285	429	20.7%	-0.17 [-0.32, -0.02]	2001
Cohen 2011 (1)	-1.065	15.0706	100	0.585	11.705	98	20.3%	-0.12 [-0.40, 0.16]	2011
Subtotal (95% CI)			378			527	41.0%	-0.16 [-0.29, -0.02]	

Heterogeneity: Tau² = 0.00; Chi² = 0.08, df = 1 (P = 0.78); I² = 0%
Test for overall effect: Z = 2.31 (P = 0.02)

Total (95% CI)			766			868	100.0%	-0.84 [-1.64, -0.03]	

Heterogeneity: Tau² = 0.80; Chi² = 191.99, df = 4 (P < 0.00001); I² = 98%
Test for overall effect: Z = 2.04 (P = 0.04)
Test for subgroup differences: Chi² = 14.50, df = 1 (P = 0.0001), I² = 93.1%
(1) Mean change for composite of SF-36 Physical and Mental Components

Economic Outcomes

Rates for hospital admissions and emergency department visits. The effect of SMAs on hospital admissions was reported in five studies.[3,14,19,26,37] Four studies reported admission rates involving 603 patients followed for 6 to 18 months. In three of these, admission rates were lower with SMAs, but the result was statistically significant in only one study.[19] The fifth study[37] followed 707 patients for 2 years and reported a statistically nonsignificant lower proportion of patients with a hospital admission who were randomized to SMAs (16.9% versus 21.0%, p=0.10).

Effects on emergency department visits were reported in the same five studies. Two studies reported significantly lower visit rates[3] or the proportion with an emergency department visit.[37] Rates were not significantly different in the other three studies. Observational studies did not report comparative effects on admission rates or emergency department visits.

Costs. Four studies reported effects on total costs, one in a large HMO,[37] two in a university-affiliated general medical clinic serving low-income patients,[14,15] and another in an Italian diabetes clinic.[20] Findings were mixed. In the largest trial testing a low-intensity intervention,[37] the total health care costs (excluding the clinical study personnel) did not differ significantly. The studies by Clancy et al.[14,15] tested more robust interventions. The earlier study found significantly higher total costs (inpatient, outpatient, and emergency department costs) for SMAs compared with usual care ($2,886 versus $1,490 per patient over six months; p=0.0003). Total costs were heavily influence by higher inpatient costs for the SMA group. In the later study, 1-year charges were significantly lower for the SMA group ($5,869 versus $8,412 per patient, p<0.05). Lower modeled charges were driven primarily by lower outpatient charges, in particular for specialty visits. The study by Trento et al.,[20] conducted in Italy, reports costs that may not be applicable to the U.S. health system. An evaluation that included staff costs, medications, and transportation costs for diabetes care showed a small increase for SMA patients ($597 versus $570 over 4 years, p=NR). Observational studies did not report comparative costs.

Effect of SMAs on Outcomes for Older Adults

Patient selection for SMA studies among older adults

Only three studies evaluated SMA interventions in older adults. Two of the four studies required a minimum age of 60; the other two used 65. All studies required some elevated use of health care in the past year; two operationalized that directly, while the third required a hospitalization in the past year.

We identified two randomized trials[9,11] that evaluated the effects of SMAs in 615 older adults with a recent hospitalization or other criteria for increased utilization. One observational study evaluated a similar population of 2251 older adults.[10] All studies were conducted in primary care, in group-model HMO settings in the United States, and compared SMAs with usual care. The mean age of participants ranged from 73.5 to 78.2 years of age. The most common chronic conditions were arthritis, hypertension, difficulty hearing, heart disease, liver disease, and bladder/kidney disease. All studies reported effects on utilization or costs at 1 year or greater. One trial was rated fair quality[11] and one poor quality;[9] the observational study was rated fair quality.[10] In the trial by Scott et al.,[11] only participants expressing a strong interest in group care (37% of those eligible) were randomized. Methodological problems included failure to describe allocation concealment, outcomes assessed without blinding to intervention, and poor specification of outcome measures. Additional study details are in Appendix G.

The design of SMA visits was similar to the diabetes studies, except that fewer disciplines participated in the clinical teams. Detailed intervention descriptions are in Appendix H.

Treatment Experience and Adherence Outcomes

All studies reported a measure of patient experience. The two trials reported patient perceptions of quality of care, and both reported higher quality ratings with SMAs compared with usual care. In the study by Beck et al.,[9] more patients rated the overall quality of care as excellent (37% versus 27%, p=0.019), and Scott et al.[11] found that patients assigned to SMAs rated the quality of care 0.3 points higher on a 1-to-4 scale than usual care patients did (p=0.048). In the observational study, only SMA participants rated satisfaction, and 90 percent of participants reported satisfaction with four aspects of group visits, including the visit overall. In aggregate, these results support high levels of satisfaction with group visits among older adults. No study evaluated staff satisfaction using a validated measure, and no study reported comparative data on medication adherence. In the study by Levine et al.,[10] 90 percent of SMA providers agreed or strongly agreed that they felt a lot of satisfaction from group visits, and 50 percent endorsed that group visits enhance their practice. Beck et al.[9] reported that participants attended 55 percent of scheduled SMA visits. Among participants with a high interest in group visits, Scott et al.[11] reported 2 or fewer visits over 24 months by approximately 25 percent of patients.

Biophysical Outcomes

Biophysical outcomes were not reported, likely because patients were selected on the basis of age and health care utilization rather than a particular illness.

Health-Related Quality-of-Life Outcomes

Both trials reported effects on overall health status (via the Likert scale) and functional status using activities of daily living or instrumental activities of daily living; there were no differences in outcomes for any of these measures. Scott et al.[11] reported effects on HRQOL using a 10-point scale with 10 indicating the highest quality of life possible. Participants randomized to SMAs rated HRQOL higher at 24-month followup (mean score, SMA 7.2 [1.8] versus usual care 6.3 [2.0]; p=0.002). The single observational study did not reported effects on HRQOL or functional status.

Economic Outcomes

Rates for hospital admissions and emergency department visits. All studies showed fewer admissions in the SMA group, but the difference was statistically significant in only one study (mean admissions/patient, 0.44 [0.89] versus 0.82 [1.7]; p=0.013).[11] SMA visits were also associated with a statistically significant decrease in emergency department visits in both trials (mean difference in visit rates/year, 0.22 to 0.26); the observational study did not report emergency department visits. Other outpatient utilization was not significantly lower in the SMA groups. Primary care visits were not lower in any of the three studies, and only one of two studies[9] found significantly lower specialty visits.

Costs. The specific approach to cost analyses varied, but all studies included estimated costs of SMA visits. Total costs were lower for the SMA group in each study (range in mean difference in annual costs, -$178 to -$1599) but varied substantially across studies and did not reach statistical significance for any study. The two trials reported lower hospital costs, ranging from -$178/person per year (p=NR) to -$1145/person per year (p=0.07); the observational study did not report hospital costs. Other cost data were not reported consistently across studies.

KEY QUESTION 2: For adults with chronic medical conditions, do the effects of SMAs vary by patient characteristics (e.g., specific chronic medical conditions and severity of disease)?

We planned to address this question using two approaches, beginning with comparing the effects of SMAs across conditions. However, studies did not examine subgroups within their populations, and there was too little variability in diagnosis across studies for analysis—all condition-specific studies enrolled patients with diabetes. The single study enrolling adults with type 1 diabetes found similar treatment effects compared with those enrolling adults with type 2 diabetes. Second, we planned and conducted an evaluation of the association between treatment effects and baseline severity of disease. This analysis was possible only for the studies enrolling patients with diabetes. We used meta-regression analysis to examine the baseline association between A1c and treatment effects on glucose control. Baseline A1c was not associated with treatment effects (B=0.14 increase in A1c per 1 point increase in baseline A1c; 95% CI, -0.47 to 0.75; p=0.66). However, this analysis is limited by the relatively small number of studies, indirect comparisons, and potential for ecological fallacy since only the average baseline A1c for the study sample was available. A more robust approach would be a meta-analysis at the patient level, where baseline A1c is evaluated for each patient; however, these data were not available.

KEY QUESTION 3: Is the intensity of the intervention or the components used by SMAs associated with intervention effects?

Characteristics of the SMA interventions are summarized in Table 3 (KQ 1). Detailed descriptions for each study are given in Appendix H. As described in the Methods section, we developed a measure of intervention robustness based on seven intervention components. Two of the components (involving a behavioral health specialist or a medication change during SMA visits) were weighted double, and thus scores could range from zero to nine. For these analyses, we limited the sample to the trials in patients with diabetes and used A1c as the outcome, yielding a set of studies with similar characteristics except for the independent variable of interest (intervention robustness). We used meta-regression analyses to examine the relationship between robustness and intervention effects on A1c. For the 12 trials, robustness scores ranged from 3 to 8 (median=5). There was no association between intervention robustness score and treatment effects (B=0.02 decrease in A1c per 1-point increase in robustness score; 95% CI, -0.30 to 0.25; p=0.88).

SUMMARY AND DISCUSSION

SMAs have the potential to offer chronic disease care that is more efficient while improving staff satisfaction and patient outcomes. We identified 15 RCTs and 4 observational studies of varying quality comparing SMAs with usual care or enhanced usual care. Studies were conducted exclusively in patients with diabetes or in older adults with higher than average medical utilization. No eligible studies enrolled patients with the other chronic conditions of interest: coronary artery disease, chronic heart failure, asthma, chronic obstructive pulmonary disease, hyperlipidemia, or hypertension. This limited diversity in patient populations compromised our ability to determine if effects varied by condition. However, the included studies reported outcomes ranging from patient experience to biophysical and economic outcomes. These findings and the overall strength of evidence are summarized and discussed by key question.

SUMMARY OF EVIDENCE BY KEY QUESTION

Key Question 1

Few studies (0 to 3) reported effects on staff experience, patient experience, or treatment adherence. The strength of evidence for each of these outcomes was judged to be insufficient to estimate an effect of the SMA intervention in both patients with diabetes and older adults.

The most robust finding of this evidence synthesis is that SMAs for patients with diabetes appear to have a significant impact on biophysical outcomes. Hemoglobin A1c improved by approximately 0.6 percentage points, and systolic blood pressure by about 5 mmHg; both these findings were statistically significant. LDL-C improved by approximately 7 mg/dl, but this was not statistically significant. While each individual finding is only moderately robust given the limitations in study quality and unexplained variability in intervention effects, the constellation of findings taken together indicates that SMAs help intermediate clinical outcomes for type 2 diabetes. Similar outcomes were not reported in older adults.

For patients with diabetes, there was significant improvement on HRQOL, measured in 3 of 4 studies with a relatively sensitive, disease-specific, quality-of-life scale. Positive effects on HRQOL were found in one trial conducted in older adults, but functional status was not affected in these studies. Studies in older adults show a pattern of lower health care utilization, but the number of studies and participants are relatively few and these results should be considered preliminary. In patients with diabetes, lower hospitalization was the most consistent effect, but effects on other economic outcomes were too preliminary to estimate an effect. Our judgments about the strength of evidence (SOE) prioritized data from RCTs.

Table 5. Summary of the intervention effects and SOE for KQ 1

| Population | Number of Studies[a] (Subjects) | Domains Pertaining to SOE | | | | SOE |
		Risk of Bias: Study Design/ Quality	Consistency	Directness	Precision	Effect Estimate (95% CI)
Staff experience						**Insufficient**
Diabetes	0	NA	NA	NA	NA	Not estimable
Older adults	1 (1236)	Obs/Fair	NA	Direct	Imprecise	Not estimable
Patient experience						**Insufficient**
Diabetes	2 (769)	RCT/Fair	Consistent	Direct	Imprecise	No effect
Older adults	2 (444)	RCT/Fair	Inconsistent	Direct	Imprecise	Small to large positive effect
Treatment adherence						**Insufficient**
Diabetes	3 (536)	RCT/Fair	Some inconsistency	Direct	Imprecise	Not estimable
Older adults	0	NA	NA	NA	NA	Not estimable
Biophysical						
Diabetes: A1c	13 (2921)	RCT/Good	Inconsistent	Direct	Some imprecision	MD = -0.55 (-0.99 to -0.11) Moderate SOE
Diabetes: Total Cholesterol	5 (1556)	RCT/Fair	Inconsistent	Direct	Imprecise	MD = -4.9 (-17.8 to 7.9) Low SOE
LDL Cholesterol	5 (997)	RCT/Fair	Inconsistent	Direct	Imprecise	MD -6.6 (-16.1 to 2.8) Low SOE
Diabetes: Blood pressure	5 (1125)	RCT/Good	Consistent	Direct	Some imprecision	MD = -5.2 (-7.4 to -3.1) Moderate SOE
Older adults	0	NA	NA	NA	NA	Not estimable
Health-related quality of life or functional status						
Diabetes	5 (1561)	RCT/Fair	Inconsistent	Direct	Imprecise	SMD = -0.84 (-1.6 to -0.03) Low SOE
Older adults	2 (615)	RCT/Fair	Inconsistent	Direct	Imprecise	Not estimable
Economic						
Diabetes	5 (1339)	RCT/Good	Inconsistent	Direct	Imprecise	*ED visits* lower rates in 2 of 5 studies Insufficient SOE
	5 (1339)	RCT/Good	Consistent	Direct	Some imprecision	*Hospitalizations* lower in 4 of 5 studies Low SOE
	4 (1125)	RCT/Fair	Inconsistent	Direct	Imprecise	*Total costs* range from lower to higher Insufficient SOE

| Population | Number of Studies[a] (Subjects) | Domains Pertaining to SOE | | | | SOE |
		Risk of Bias: Study Design/ Quality	Consistency	Directness	Precision	Effect Estimate (95% CI)
Older adults	2 (615)	RCT/Fair	Consistent	Direct	Imprecise	*ED visits* lower rates in 2 of 2 studies Low SOE
	2 (615)	RCT/Fair	Some inconsistency	Direct	Imprecise	*Hospitalizations* lower in 1 of 2 studies Insufficient SOE
	2 (615)	RCT/Fair	Inconsistent	Direct	Imprecise	*Total costs* lower but not statistically significant Insufficient SOE

[a]Studies (subjects) given are for randomized trials; observational studies were also considered in SOE ratings but are not listed separately in the table.

Abbreviations: CI=confidence interval; ED=emergency department; MD=mean difference; NA=not applicable; RCT=randomized controlled trial; RD=risk difference; RR=risk ratio; SMD=standardized mean difference; SOE=strength of evidence

Key Questions 2 and 3

No studies explored KQ 2 (identifying the subgroups of patients that would benefit most from an SMA intervention) or KQ 3 (identifying the specific components of an SMA intervention that were most potent). We devised a robustness score to attempt to address KQ 3, but it was not able to discriminate degrees of effectiveness among intervention components. More than 70 percent of all studies were similar on six of the seven variables used in the robustness score: (1) whether the team was continuous, (2) whether the group was closed, (3) whether individual breakout sessions were conducted, (4) whether medication changes were made, (5) how long each session was, and (6) whether there was contact outside the session. It is possible that there are other more important variables that are not being measured with current approaches. The strength of evidence for both questions was judged to be insufficient.

CLINICAL AND POLICY IMPLICATIONS

A key finding is that SMAs have been evaluated primarily in patients with diabetes, and to a lesser extent and with a narrow range of outcomes for older adults with high utilization. Even where the data are more robust in those with diabetes, it is challenging to place into context the improvements seen in biophysical parameters with SMAs. However, we can discuss the clinical importance of these findings in at least two ways. First, we can compare the results to clinical trial data relative to starting any agent for these conditions. The improvement seen in one year on systolic blood pressure across all arms of the Antihypertensive and Lipid-Lowering Treatment to Prevent Heart Attack Trial (ALLHAT), trial, after adding the chosen first medication, was approximately 6.6 mmHg; patients in SMAs achieved approximately 75 percent of that level of improvement.[38] Similarly, adding a first-line oral hypoglycemic agent at a maximally tolerated dose usually lowers A1c by 1 to 1.5 percentage points;[38] patients in SMAs achieve 33 to 50 percent of that goal. The change in LDL-C of 7 mg/dl is much smaller compared with drug effect, approximately 15 percent of what would be expected with clinical trial doses of an HMG-CoA reductase inhibitor ("statin"). However, each drug comparison is made relative to placebo controls. For SMA interventions, the comparator is usual care, which typically includes medication treatment, and thus one would expect the effects to be smaller.

Another way to evaluate the improvements observed with SMA is against the known standard deviations for the outcomes in the population of patients with disease, and then calculate effect sizes. While many different values for standard deviations for the relevant parameters are reported in the literature, effect sizes of SMA interventions for systolic BP, A1c, and LDL-C are approximately 0.5, 0.33, and 0.25, respectively. These are considered moderate to small effect sizes, but all would be considered important.[39]

The improvements in A1c and blood pressure, and the more modest improvement in LDL-C are possibly synergistic, or at least additive, in prevention of the macrovascular and microvascular complications of diabetes.[40] Thus, as a whole, SMAs may impact the risk of complications among patients with diabetes. Even if half the effect were lost in translation due to lower treatment fidelity when implemented outside of clinical trials, there would still likely be an important improvement in complication risk for patients enrolled in a diabetes SMA intervention. However, it is important to remember that the degree of synergy in the context of improvements in multiple outcomes is guesswork at best; SMAs—and indeed multicomponent health services in general—have not been studied with enough patients to determine their actual effects on major cardiovascular or microvascular complications.

Finally, many authors propose that SMAs are more satisfying than standard outpatient visits for both patients and providers, but few have measured patient and staff satisfaction. Because SMAs are a major shift in clinic organization, more data are needed on these variables as well as cost-to-benefit ratios before a general policy recommendation can be made.

Generalizability of Findings

The results of the diabetes studies have limitations to their external validity. Using the PICOTS framework (population, intervention, comparator, outcome, timing, setting), the applicability of the findings appears strong with respect to (1) population because a reasonable balance of race and sex was achieved among patients, (2) outcomes because there is general consensus that A1c, blood pressure, and LDL-C are the important outcomes in diabetes, and (3) timeframes because there is general consensus that improvement of 6 months or longer is clinically relevant. However, none of the studies examined maintenance of effect after the intervention ended. Although similar in many aspects, there were enough differences in intervention process that a conclusion as to what makes an SMA intervention particularly successful could not be drawn. In addition, what constituted usual care was inconsistently defined. Therefore, intervention heterogeneity and the types of usual care comparators, may also be important limitations to the generalizability of our results.

The heterogeneity of the studies is concerning. Complex health services interventions are often a black box; that is, they contain many components that are hard to capture and tease out even in a well-conducted analysis. If there was a particular aspect of these interventions that was critical to predicting improved clinical outcomes, we were unable to capture that with the available data. This raises the question of a possible uncaptured element of SMAs that is important for potency, effectiveness, or generalizability. Without further, more mechanistic studies that attempt to elucidate the key components of an SMA intervention, implementation of a diabetes SMA or design of an SMA for another condition will be at least partially based on reasoned judgment rather than strict evidence-based decision making.

An additional concern is that none of these studies was conducted in "real world" settings. All of the diabetes studies were conducted in academic, government, or vertically integrated systems. There are two potential reasons for this. First, all complex chronic care redesign interventions are easier to implement in systems that are either highly controlled or in which there is interest in research. Second, SMAs are difficult to implement in fee-for-service, independent clinics because they are unlikely to derive any financial benefits from improved quality of care but would have to absorb the cost in time and money of implementing the SMA. It is possible that this barrier could be relieved by Accountable Care Organizations, but this theory is still untested. Lastly, academic, government, or vertically integrated systems may also have very high quality usual care. While factors related to setting may not negatively impact the generalizability of these results for implementation of diabetes or other SMAs within vertically integrated systems such as the VA, they do suggest caution when considering the use of SMAs outside such systems.

Should SMAs Be Implemented?

The clearest finding of this evidence synthesis is that the existing knowledge base does not provide enough evidence to make a strictly evidence-driven decision about implementation of SMAs in any context except diabetes. Regarding diabetes SMA implementation, this evidence synthesis raises several key issues summarized in Table 6.

Table 6. Implementation issues

Issue for Implementation of Diabetes SMAs	Potential Solution
Enrollment There was no clear indication of which patients will receive the most benefit from this alternative structure.	Allow selection criteria for SMAs to fit specific local needs.

Elements of intervention
 	
There was no clear indication of which elements were most effective.
	Use the most prevalent common elements:
	    Prescribing clinician
	    A consistent clinical lead for the SMA group
	    At least 3 team members
	    Closed group participants
	    Individual time with clinician (brief)
	    Medications evaluated
	    Group duration of 90 to 120 minutes
	
	Variable elements that could be tailored to clinic or patient population:
	    Group size
	    Participation of family and friends
	    Contact with participants outside of group

Potential mechanisms of intervention Very few studies reported any intermediate or mechanistic outcomes such as self-management, medication change, or access to care.	Measure these at implementation; use Plan-Do-Study-Act approach to allow these factors to change intervention over time.

Issue for Implementation of Diabetes SMAs	Potential Solution
Infrastructure changes There was no clear indication whether the change in clinic structure was more effective or efficient.	In already vertically integrated settings, such as VA, these changes are not as difficult. The broad-based improvement seen was clinically meaningful balanced against satisfaction and cost, especially for older adults.

SMAs also have costs. These costs are not just the labor cost of redirecting providers away from their existing clinical responsibilities to conduct an SMA; there is also the time and labor cost to establish a new structure for care. This lack of information about both direct costs and changes in utilization in all but older adults who are high utilizers of the health care system is a key gap in the existing literature. For those patients, hospital admissions, ER visits and total costs were consistently lower with SMAs. Also, implementation of SMAs will not succeed if either patients or providers are unsatisfied with the new structure, and effects on patient and staff experience remain largely unknown, again with the exception of older adults who expressed increased satisfaction with SMAs.

STRENGTHS AND LIMITATIONS

Our study has a number of strengths, including a protocol-driven review, a comprehensive search, careful quality assessment, and rigorous quantitative synthesis methods. Our report, and the literature, also has limitations. An important limitation is the lack of breadth to the types of patients and illnesses that have been studied in the context of an SMA. The evidence synthesis found no explicit data regarding system-level, as opposed to patient-level, benefits of SMAs; the fact that as many studies viewed the SMA as an add-on to, rather than a replacement for, usual primary care suggests that improvements in access may not be as great as desired. In addition, the components of the interventions were often not described adequately for replication, especially the content of the group education time. Finally, outcomes reported varied substantially across studies and our attempts to explain the observed variability in intervention effects were unsuccessful. With unexplained variability, summary measures of treatment effect may not adequately describe the expected effects of the intervention.

RECOMMENDATIONS FOR FUTURE RESEARCH

We used the framework recommended Robinson et al.[41] to identify gaps in evidence and classify why these gaps exist (Table 7). The next generation of research in SMAs for patients with diabetes and other conditions should close the gaps outlined in the previous section.

Table 7. Evidence gaps and future research

Evidence Gap	Reason	Type of Studies to Consider
Patients		
Absence of data for patients with conditions other than diabetes mellitus and high utilization	Insufficient information	Single and multisite RCTs Quasi-experimental studies
Interventions		

Evidence Gap	Reason	Type of Studies to Consider
Uncertain which elements of an SMA intervention are most effective and efficient	Insufficient information	RCTs of head-to-head comparisons of different types of SMAs; Disaggregation trials
Outcomes		
Uncertain effects on patient and staff satisfaction	Insufficient information	Nonrandomized or cluster randomized, multisite implementation studies, qualitative studies
Uncertain effects on physiological variables other than HbA1c	Insufficient information	Large scale RCTs Nonrandomized, cluster controlled trials, controlled before-and-after studies, interrupted time series
Uncertain effects on health system costs with the exception of the elderly high utilizers of the health system	Insufficient information	Costs analyses
Uncertain whether there would be unintended consequences to other aspects of the health care system if SMAs were implemented	Insufficient information	Multisite observational studies

Abbreviation: RCT=randomized controlled trial

Our review shows that SMAs, typically using closed panels with individual breakouts and the opportunity for medication management, help intermediate clinical outcomes for type 2 diabetes. A smaller literature shows positive effects on patient experience in older adults and the possibility of lower health care utilization. SMAs may be most effective for illnesses such as diabetes that have a phase in which the risk of complication is relatively high while the disease is simultaneously asymptomatic, and in which medication titration and self-management are important. Until further studies are done that allow for comparisons across conditions, the targeting of SMA for chronic conditions other than diabetes will remain speculative. Finally, repeating the existing diabetes SMA efficacy trials in fee-for-service settings would be important to understand the extent to which SMAs work when the profit motive is essential to the practice model.

REFERENCES

1.   Fletcher RD, Amdur RL, Kolodner R, et al. Blood Pressure Control Among US Veterans: A Large Multi-Year Analysis of Blood Pressure Data from the VA Health Data Repository. *Circulation.* 2012.

2.   King H, Aubert RE, Herman WH. Global burden of diabetes, 1995-2025: prevalence, numerical estimates, and projections. *Diabetes Care.* 1998;21(9):1414-31.

3.   Edelman D, Fredrickson SK, Melnyk SD, et al. Medical clinics versus usual care for patients with both diabetes and hypertension: a randomized trial. *Ann Intern Med.* 2010;152(11):689-96.

4.   Jaber R, Braksmajer A, Trilling JS. Group visits: A qualitative review of current research. *Journal of the American Board of Family Medicine.* 2006;19(3):276-290.

5.   Kirsh S, Watts S, Pascuzzi K, et al. Shared medical appointments based on the chronic care model: a quality improvement project to address the challenges of patients with diabetes with high cardiovascular risk. *Qual Saf Health Care.* 2007;16(5):349-53.

6.   Noffsinger E. Increasing quality care and access while reducing cost through drop-in group medical appointments (DIGMAs). *Group Pract J.* 1999;48(1):12-18.

7.   Riley SB, Marshall ES. Group visits in diabetes care: a systematic review. *Diabetes Educ.* 2010;36(6):936-44.

8.   Taveira TH, Friedmann PD, Cohen LB, et al. Pharmacist-led group medical appointment model in type 2 diabetes. *Diabetes Educ.* 2010;36(1):109-17.

9.   Beck A, Scott J, Williams P, et al. A randomized trial of group outpatient visits for chronically ill older HMO members: the Cooperative Health Care Clinic. *J Am Geriatr Soc.* 1997;45(5):543-9.

10. Levine MD, Ross TR, Balderson BH, et al. Implementing group medical visits for older adults at group health cooperative. *J Am Geriatr Soc.* 2010;58(1):168-72.

11. Scott JC, Conner DA, Venohr I, et al. Effectiveness of a group outpatient visit model for chronically ill older health maintenance organization members: a 2-year randomized trial of the cooperative health care clinic. *J Am Geriatr Soc.* 2004;52(9):1463-70.

12. Coleman EA, Eilertsen TB, Kramer AM, et al. Reducing emergency visits in older adults with chronic illness. A randomized, controlled trial of group visits. *Eff Clin Pract.* 2001;4(2):49-57.

13. Bray P, Thompson D, Wynn JD, et al. Confronting disparities in diabetes care: the clinical effectiveness of redesigning care management for minority patients in rural primary care practices. *J Rural Health.* 2005;21(4):317-21.

14. Clancy DE, Cope DW, Magruder KM, et al. Evaluating concordance to American Diabetes Association standards of care for type 2 diabetes through group visits in an uninsured or inadequately insured patient population. *Diabetes Care.* 2003;26(7):2032-6.

15. Clancy DE, Huang P, Okonofua E, et al. Group visits: promoting adherence to diabetes guidelines. *J Gen Intern Med.* 2007;22(5):620-4.

16. Culhane-Pera K, Peterson KA, Crain AL, et al. Group visits for Hmong adults with type 2 diabetes mellitus: a pre-post analysis. *J Health Care Poor Underserved.* 2005;16(2):315-27.

17. Gutierrez N, Gimple NE, Dallo FJ, et al. Shared medical appointments in a residency clinic: an exploratory study among Hispanics with diabetes. *Am J Manag Care.* 2011;17(6 Spec No.):e212-4.

18. Naik AD, Palmer N, Petersen NJ, et al. Comparative effectiveness of goal setting in diabetes mellitus group clinics: randomized clinical trial. *Arch Intern Med.* 2011;171(5):453-9.

19. Sadur CN, Moline N, Costa M, et al. Diabetes management in a health maintenance organization. Efficacy of care management using cluster visits. *Diabetes Care.* 1999;22(12):2011-7.

20. Trento M, Passera P, Tomalino M, et al. Group visits improve metabolic control in type 2 diabetes: a 2-year follow-up. *Diabetes Care.* 2001;24(6):995-1000.

21. Trento M, Passera P, Borgo E, et al. A 3-year prospective randomized controlled clinical trial of group care in type 1 diabetes. *Nutr Metab Cardiovasc Dis.* 2005;15(4):293-301.

22. Trento M, Gamba S, Gentile L, et al. Rethink Organization to iMprove Education and Outcomes (ROMEO): a multicenter randomized trial of lifestyle intervention by group care to manage type 2 diabetes. *Diabetes Care.* 2010;33(4):745-7.

23. Krzywkowski-Mohn SM. Diabetic control and patient perception of the scheduled in group medical appointment at the Cincinnati Veterans Administration Medical Center. ProQuest Information & Learning; 2009.

24. Moher D, Liberati A, Tetzlaff J, et al. Preferred reporting items for systematic reviews and meta-analyses: the PRISMA statement. *PLoS Med.* 2009;6(7):e1000097.

25. Wilczynski NL, McKibbon KA, Haynes RB. Response to Glanville et al.: How to identify randomized controlled trials in MEDLINE: ten years on. *J Med Libr Assoc.* 2007;95(2):117-8; author reply 119-20.

26. Taveira TH, Dooley AG, Cohen LB, et al. Pharmacist-led group medical appointments for the management of type 2 diabetes with comorbid depression in older adults. *Ann Pharmacother.* 2011;45(11):1346-55.

27. Loney-Hutchinson LM, Provilus AD, Jean-Louis G, et al. Group visits in the management of diabetes and hypertension: effect on glycemic and blood pressure control. *Current Diabetes Reports.* 2009;9(3):238-242.

28. Kirsh SR, Aron DC. Integrating the chronic-care model and the ACGME competencies: using shared medical appointments to focus on systems-based practice... Accreditation Council for Graduate Medical Education. *Quality & Safety in Health Care.* 2008;17(1):15-19.

29.   Agency for Healthcare Research and Quality. Methods Guide for Effectiveness and Comparative Effectiveness Reviews. Rockville, MD: Agency for Healthcare Research and Quality. Available at: http://www.effectivehealthcare.ahrq.gov/index.cfm/search-for-guides-reviews-and-reports/?pageaction=displayproduct&productid=318. Accessed May 10, 2012.

30.   Viswanathan M, Berkman ND. Development of the RTI Item Bank on Risk of Bias and Precision of Observational Studies. Methods Research Report. (Prepared by the RTI International-University of North Carolina Evidence-based Practice Center under Contract No. 290-2007-0056-I.) AHRQ Publication No. 11-EHC028-EF. Rockville, MD: Agency for Healthcare Research and Quality. Available at: http://www.effectivehealthcare.ahrq.gov/ehc/products/350/784/RTI-Risk-of-Bias_Final-Report_20110916.pdf. Accessed May 15, 2012.

31.   Higgins JP, Thompson SG. Quantifying heterogeneity in a meta-analysis. *Stat Med*. 2002;21(11):1539-58.

32.   Guyatt GH, Oxman AD, Kunz R, et al. GRADE guidelines 6. Rating the quality of evidence--imprecision. *J Clin Epidemiol*. 2011;64(12):1283-93.

33.   Schunemann HJ, Oxman AD, Brozek J, et al. Grading quality of evidence and strength of recommendations for diagnostic tests and strategies. *BMJ*. 2008;336(7653):1106-10.

34.   Egger M, Davey Smith G, Schneider M, et al. Bias in meta-analysis detected by a simple, graphical test. *BMJ*. 1997;315(7109):629-34.

35.   Sterne JA, Egger M, Smith GD. Systematic reviews in health care: Investigating and dealing with publication and other biases in meta-analysis. *BMJ*. 2001;323(7304):101-5.

36.   Cohen LB, Taveira TH, Khatana SA, et al. Pharmacist-led shared medical appointments for multiple cardiovascular risk reduction in patients with type 2 diabetes. *Diabetes Educ*. 2011;37(6):801-12.

37.   Wagner EH, Grothaus LC, Sandhu N, et al. Chronic care clinics for diabetes in primary care: a system-wide randomized trial. *Diabetes Care*. 2001;24(4):695-700.

38.   Fowler MJ. Diabetes Treatment, Part 2:Oral Agents for Glycemic Management. Clinical Diabetes. October 2007 vol. 25 no. 4 131-134.

39.   Cohen J. *Statistical Power Analysis for the Behavioral Sciences (second ed.)*. Hillsdale, NJ: Lawrence Erlbaum Associates; 1988.

40.   Sehestedt T, Hansen TW, Li Y, et al. Are blood pressure and diabetes additive or synergistic risk factors? Outcome in 8494 subjects randomly recruited from 10 populations. *Hypertens Res*. 2011;34(6):714-21.

41.   Robinson KA, Saldanha IJ, Mckoy NA. Frameworks for Determining Research Gaps During Systematic Reviews. Methods Future Research Needs Report No. 2. (Prepared by the Johns Hopkins University Evidence-based Practice Center under Contract No. HHSA 290-2007-10061-I.) AHRQ Publication No. 11-EHC043-EF. Rockville, MD: Agency for Healthcare Research and Quality. June 2011. Available at: www.effectivehealthcare.ahrq.gov/reports/final.cfm. Accessed May 22, 2012.

APPENDIX A. SEARCH STRATEGIES

Table A-1. Search strategy for RCTs and observational studies (PubMed, April 2012)

Step	Category	Terms	Result
1	Terms for "group appointment"	(visit[ti] OR visits[ti] OR appointment[ti] OR appointments[ti] OR clinic[ti] OR clinics[ti] OR "Appointments and Schedules"[Mesh]) AND (group[ti] OR shared[ti] OR cluster[ti])	744
2	Terms for "shared visits"	("shared medical appointment"[tiab] OR "shared medical appointments"[tiab] OR "group care"[tiab] OR "group medical appointment"[tiab] OR "group medical appointments"[tiab] OR "cluster visit"[tiab] OR "cluster visits"[tiab] OR "group visit"[tiab] OR "group visits"[tiab] OR "shared medical visit"[tiab] OR "shared medical visits"[tiab] OR "group medical clinic"[tiab] OR "group medical clinics"[tiab])	313
3	Combined intervention terms	#1 OR #2	961
4	Terms for RCT study design	(randomized controlled trial[pt] OR controlled clinical trial[pt] OR randomized[tiab] OR randomised[tiab] OR randomization[tiab] OR randomisation[tiab] OR placebo[tiab] OR drug therapy[sh] OR randomly[tiab] OR trial[tiab] OR groups[tiab] OR Clinical trial[pt] OR "clinical trial"[tw] OR "clinical trials"[tw] OR "evaluation studies"[Publication Type] OR "evaluation studies as topic"[MeSH Terms] OR "evaluation study"[tw] OR evaluation studies[tw] OR "intervention studies"[MeSH Terms] OR "intervention study"[tw] OR "intervention studies"[tw] OR "cohort studies"[MeSH Terms] OR cohort[tw] OR "longitudinal studies"[MeSH Terms] OR "longitudinal"[tw] OR longitudinally[tw] OR "prospective"[tw] OR prospectively[tw] OR "follow up"[tw] OR "comparative study"[Publication Type] OR "comparative study"[tw] OR systematic[subset] OR "meta-analysis"[Publication Type] OR "meta-analysis as topic"[MeSH Terms] OR "meta-analysis"[tw] OR "meta-analyses"[tw]) NOT (Editorial[ptyp] OR Letter[ptyp] OR Case Reports[ptyp] OR Comment[ptyp]) NOT (animals[mh] NOT humans[mh])	4216173
5	Intervention AND RCT	#3 AND #4	466
6	Terms for observational studies	"pre-post"[tiab] OR "post-test"[tiab] OR "post test"[tiab] OR pretest[tiab] OR pre-test[tiab] OR "pre test"[tiab] OR quasi-experiment*[tiab] OR quasiexperiment*[tiab] OR quasirandom*[tiab] OR quasi-random*[tiab] OR quasi-control*[tiab] OR quasicontrol*[tiab] OR ("time series"[tiab] AND interrupt[tiab]) OR ("time points"[tiab] AND (multiple[tiab] OR one[tiab] OR two[tiab] OR three[tiab] OR four[tiab] OR five[tiab] OR six[tiab] OR seven[tiab] OR eight[tiab] OR nine[tiab] OR ten[tiab] OR month*[tiab] OR day*[tiab] OR week*[tiab] OR hour*[tiab])) OR (before[tiab] AND after[tiab]) OR (*before[tiab] AND during[tiab])	44225
7	Intervention and Observational	#3 AND #6	11
8	Applies limits to combined RCT and observational studies	#5 OR #7 with limits: English, Publication Date from 1996 to 2011	323

APPENDIX B. EXCLUDED STUDIES

All articles listed below were reviewed in their full-text version and excluded for the reason indicated. An alphabetical reference list follows the table.

Table B-1. Excluded studies with reasons

Reference	Not full publication, peer-reviewed, or primary data	Not study population of interest	Not eligible study design	Comparator not of interest	Intervention does not meet protocol definition	Not an outcome of interest reported at ≥3 months
AHRQ, 2003 (943)	X					
AHRQ, 2007 (844)	X					
Anonymous, 1996 (946)	X					
Anonymous, 2001 (913)	X					
Anonymous, 2001 (944)	X					
Anonymous, 2003 (351)	X					
Antonucci, 2008 (835)	X					
Barud, 2006 (730)			X			
Block, 2010 (747)	X					
Bray, 2005 (299)			X			
Bronson, 2004 (1331)			X			
Brooks, 2007 (265)			X			
Campbell, 2007 (518)		X				
Clancy, 2003 (347)						X
Clancy, 2007 (259)						X
Conrad, 2008 (775)		X				
Desouza, 2010 (157)			X			
Anonymous, 2001 (373)	X					
Dontje, 2011 (607)			X			
Falck-Ytter, 2009 (1286)	X					
Geller, 2011 (142)			X			
Harris, 2010 (178)		X				
Jaber, 2006 (780)	X					
Jeanfreau, 2008 (732)	X					
Anonymous, 2002 (955)	X					
Katz, 1975 (596)	X					
Kirsh, 2006 (1312)	X					
Krywkowski-Mohn, 2009 (1508)	X					
Lin, 2008 (214)			X			
Loney-Hutchinson, 2009 (703)			X			
Mackay, 2011 (649)		X				
Masley, 2001 (386)					X	
Mayo Clinic Proceedings, 2008 (507)					X	
McCulloch, 1998 (410)			X			
McHugh, 1998 (420)					X	
Miller, 329 (329)			X			
Murray, 2005 (313)	X					
Ostroff, 2010 (1278)	X					
Palaniappan, 2011 (135)		X				
Peterson, 2007 (929)	X					
Porta, 2004 (326)						X
Reiber, 2004 (328)					X	

Reference	Not full publication, peer-reviewed, or primary data	Not study population of interest	Not eligible study design	Comparator not of interest	Intervention does not meet protocol definition	Not an outcome of interest reported at ≥3 months
Rivard, 2009 (498)	X					
Rossi, 2011 (1269)	X					
Salinas, 2006 (1308)	X					
Salinas-Martinez, 2009 (1282)	X					
Sanchez, 2011 (608)			X			
Scott, 1998 (426)	X					
Shahady, 2008 (795)	X					
Shahady, 2010 (465)	X					
Stoner, 2001 (375)					X	
Taveira, 2008 (1686)			X			
Thompson, 2000 (875)	X					
Thompson, 2001 (389)		X				
Trento, 2006 (291)						X
Trento, 2008 (1291)	X					
Trento, 2008 (238)						X
Trento, 2009 (1283)	X					
Trento, 2009 (1284)	X					
Trento, 2009 (904)				X		
Vachon, 2007 (237)			X			
Vinci, 2006 (1311)	X					
Watkinson, 2004 (976)	X					
Watts, 2009 (1582)			X			
Weber, 2004 (1333)	X					
Westheimer, 2009 (666)			X			
Wheelock, 2009 (211)			X			
Worth, 1990 (557)					X	
Yehle, 2007 (689)	X					
Yehle, 2009 (213)						X
Yu, 2010 (165)					X	

LIST OF EXCLUDED STUDIES

Agency for Healthcare Research and Quality. Group visits to primary care doctors by disadvantaged diabetes patients result in better diabetes care than individual visits. *AHRQ Research Activities*. 2003(278):14-14.

Agency for Healthcare Research and Quality. Studies examine medication adherence and group medical visits among persons with high blood pressure. *AHRQ Research Activities*. 2007(326):16-17.

Anonymous. Colorado HMO trades traditional doctor visits for group clinics. *Disease State Management*. 1996;2(2):13-17.

Anonymous. DIGMAs (drop-in group medical appointments): satisfaction Rx for doctors and patients. *Hosp Peer Rev*. 2001;26(6):81-2.

Anonymous. Researchers find new value in group visit concept among chronically ill adults. *Disease Management Advisor*. 2001;7(8):121-125.

Anonymous. Take steps to ensure group visits are successful: start with chronic patient groups. *Patient Education Management*. 2001;8(8):92.

Anonymous. Group appointments for seniors continue to prove their worth. *Senior Care Management*. 2002;5(4):57-59.

Anonymous. Shared medical appointments save money for capitated groups. *Capitation Manag Rep*. 2003;10(2):20-4, 17.

Antonucci J. A new approach to group visits: helping high-need patients make behavioral change. *Fam Pract Manag*. 2008;15(4):A6-8.

Barud S, Marcy T, Armor B, et al. Development and implementation of group medical visits at a family medicine center. *Am J Health Syst Pharm*. 2006;63(15):1448-1452.

Block JP. Outcomes research in review. Group visits for the treatment of hypertension among diabetics: success without a pill? *Journal of Clinical Outcomes Management*. 2010;17(8):343.

Bray P, Roupe M, Young S, et al. Feasibility and effectiveness of system redesign for diabetes care management in rural areas: the eastern North Carolina experience. *Diabetes Educ*. 2005;31(5):712-8.

Bronson DL, Maxwell RA. Shared medical appointments. Increasing patient access without increasing physician hours. *Cleve Clin J Med*. 2004;71(5):369-+.

Brooks AD, Rihani RS, Derus CL. Pharmacist membership in a medical group's diabetes health management program. *Am J Health Syst Pharm*. 2007;64(6):617-21.

Campbell BB, Gosselin D. High patient satisfaction amongst males participating in men's educational group appointments (MEGA) for routine physical exams. *Journal of Men's Health and Gender*. 2007;4(3):266-270.

Clancy DE, Cope DW, Magruder KM, et al. Evaluating group visits in an uninsured or inadequately insured patient population with uncontrolled type 2 diabetes. *Diabetes Educ*. 2003;29(2):292-302.

Clancy DE, Yeager DE, Huang P, et al. Further evaluating the acceptability of group visits in an uninsured or inadequately insured patient population with uncontrolled type 2 diabetes. *Diabetes Educ*. 2007;33(2):309-14.

Conrad D, Fishman P, Grembowski D, et al. Access intervention in an integrated, prepaid group practice: effects on primary care physician productivity. *Health Serv Res*. 2008;43(5 Part 2):1888-1905.

Desouza CV, Rentschler L, Haynatzki G. The effect of group clinics in the control of diabetes. *Prim Care Diabetes*. 2010;4(4):251-4.

Dontje K, Forrest K. Implementing Group Visits: Are They Effective to Improve Diabetes Self-Management Outcomes? *Journal for Nurse Practitioners*. 2011;7(7):571-577.

Falck-Ytter CD, Ellert R, Denise K, et al. Effect of a Diabetes Group Clinic Using Shared Medical Visits on Outcomes for Diabetic Patients Cared for in an Urban Resident Clinic. *J Gen Intern Med*. 2009;24:252-252.

Geller JS, Orkaby A, Cleghorn GD. Impact of a group medical visit program on Latino health-related quality of life. *Explore (NY)*. 2011;7(2):94-9.

Harris MD. Shared medical appointments after cardiac surgery-the process of implementing a novel pilot paradigm to enhance comprehensive postdischarge care. *J Cardiovasc Nurs*. 2010;25(2):124-9.

Jaber J, Braksmajer A, Trilling J. Group Visits for Chronic Illness Care: Models, Benefits and Challenges. *Fam Pract Manag*. 2006;13(1):37-40.

Jeanfreau S. Group visit intervention to improve diabetes care -- a program utilizing group visits led by a nurse practitioner to improve outcomes for the medically underserved in diabetes care. *Southern Online Journal of Nursing Research*. 2008;8(2):2p.

Katz G, Hollander FL. From clinic to group practice. *Hospitals*. 1975;49(5):67-71.

Kirsh S, Watts S, Aron D, et al. Integrating residency training and diabetes shared medical appointments. *J Gen Intern Med*. 2006;21:74-75.

Krzywkowski-Mohn SM. Diabetic control and patient perception of the scheduled in group medical appointment at the Cincinnati veterans administration medical center. ProQuest Information & Learning; 2009.

Lin A, Cavendish J, Boren D, et al. A pilot study: reports of benefits from a 6-month, multidisciplinary, shared medical appointment approach for heart failure patients. *Mil Med*. 2008;173(12):1210-3.

Loney-Hutchinson LM, Provilus AD, Jean-Louis G, et al. Group visits in the management of diabetes and hypertension: effect on glycemic and blood pressure control. *Current Diabetes Reports*. 2009;9(3):238-242.

Mackay FD. Well Woman's Group Medical Appointment: For screening and preventive care. *Can Fam Physician*. 2011;57(4):e125-7.

Masley S, Phillips S, Copeland JR. Group office visits change dietary habits of patients with coronary artery disease-the dietary intervention and evaluation trial (D.I.E.T.). *J Fam Pract*. 2001;50(3):235-9.

Mayo Clinic Proceedings. Chronic care model and shared care in diabetes: Randomized trial of an electronic decision support system (Mayo Clinic Proceedings (2008) 83, 7, (747-757)). *Mayo Clin Proc*. 2008;83(10):1189.

McCulloch DK, Price MJ, Hindmarsh M, et al. A population-based approach to diabetes management in a primary care setting: early results and lessons learned. *Eff Clin Pract*. 1998;1(1):12-22.

McHugh F, Lindsay G. A study of nurse-led shared care for coronary patients. *Nurs Stand*. 1998;12(45):33.

Miller D, Zantop V, Hammer H, et al. Group medical visits for low-income women with chronic disease: a feasibility study. *J Womens Health (Larchmt)*. 2004;13(2):217-25.

Murray JL, Everson K. Group medical visits and lifestyle modifications. *J Fam Pract*. 2005;54(1):64.

Ostroff ABM, Sundel S, Bradley S, et al. Group Visits: A Model to Improve Patient Self-Management in Geriatric Ambulatory Practice. *J Am Geriatr Soc*. 2010;58:228-228.

Palaniappan LP, Muzaffar AL, Wang EJ, et al. Shared medical appointments: promoting weight loss in a clinical setting. *J Am Board Fam Med*. 2011;24(3):326-8.

Peterson C, Chicano K, Capone-Swearer D, et al. Shared medical appointments. *Nurse Practitioner World News*. 2007;12(6):16-16.

Porta M, Trento M. ROMEO: rethink organization to improve education and outcomes. *Diabet Med*. 2004;21(6):644-5.

Reiber GE, Au D, McDonell M, et al. Diabetes quality improvement in Department of Veterans Affairs Ambulatory Care Clinics: a group-randomized clinical trial. *Diabetes Care*. 2004;27 Suppl 2:B61-8.

Rivard L, Walker C, Arias A, et al. Group medical visits achieve improvements of clinical outcomes in diverse ethnic, underinsured populations: A project dulce(trademark) disease management intervention. *Diabetes*. 2009;58.

Rossi AM, Tucker AL, Hedelt AC. Cardiovascular Disease Prevention Tailored for Women: Shared Medical Appointments. *J Cardiovasc Nurs*. 2011;26(4):276-277.

Salinas AM, Irizar JF, Garza MG, et al. The cluster visit along with all-inclusive management: A good plan for improving diabetes primary care effectiveness? *Diabetes*. 2006;55:A552-A552.

Salinas-Martinez AM, Garza-Sagastegui MG, Cobos-Cruz R, et al. Effects of incorporating group visits on the metabolic control of type 2 diabetic patients. *Rev Med Chil*. 2009;137(10):1323-1332.

Sanchez I. Implementation of a Diabetes Self-management Education Program in Primary Care for Adults Using Shared Medical Appointments. *Diabetes Educ*. 2011;37(3):381-391.

Scott J, Gade G, McKenzie M, et al. Cooperative health care clinics: a group approach to individual care. *Geriatrics*. 1998;53(5):68-70, 76-8, 81; quiz 82.

Shahady EJ. Diabetes management: an approach that improves outcomes and reduces costs. *Consultant (00107069)*. 2008;48(4):331.

Shahady EJ. Group visits for diabetes: An innovative way to overcome barriers and achieve quality care. *Cons_ltant*. 2010;50(11).

Stoner KL, Lasar NJ, Butcher MK, et al. Improving glycemic control: can techniques used in a managed care setting be successfully adapted to a rural fee-for-service practice? *Am J Med Qual*. 2001;16(3):93-8.

41

Taveira TH, Pirraglia PA, Cohen LB, Wu WC. Efficacy of a pharmacist-led cardiovascular risk reduction clinic for diabetic patients with and without mental health conditions. *Prev Cardiol* 2008 Fall;11(4):195-200.

Thompson E. Physicians. The power of group visits: improved quality of care, increased productivity entice physicians to see up to 15 patients at a time. *Mod Healthc*. 2000;30(23):54.

Thompson M, Gee S, Larson P, et al. Health and loyalty promotion visits for new enrollees: results of a randomized controlled trial. *Patient Educ Couns*. 2001;42(1):53-65.

Trento M. ROMEO (Rethink Organization to iMprove Education and Outcomes). A 4-year multicentre randomised controlled trial of group care for the management of type 2 diabetes. *Diabetologia*. 2008;51:S69-S69.

Trento M, Passera P, Bajardi M, et al. Lifestyle intervention by group care prevents deterioration of Type II diabetes: a 4-year randomized controlled clinical trial. *Diab tologia*. 2002;45(9):1231-9.

Trento M, Passera P, Miselli V, et al. Evaluation of the locus of control in patients with type 2 diabetes after long-term management by group care. *Diabetes Metab*. 2006;32(1):77-81.

Trento M, Porta M. Romeo (Rethink Organization to Improve Education and Outcomes). A 4-Year Multicentre Randomised Controlled Trial of Group Care for the Management of Type 2 Diabetes. *Atherosclerosis Supplements*. 2009;10(2).

Trento M, Sicuro J, Semperbene L, et al. Cost-efficacy of group care in the management of type 2 diabetes. Economic evaluation of the ROMEO (Rethink Organization to iMprove Education and Outcomes) data set. *Diabetologia*. 2009;52:S391-S391.

Trento M, Tomelini M, Basile M, et al. The locus of control in patients with Type 1 and Type 2 diabetes managed by individual and group care. *Diabet Med*. 2008;25(1):86-90.

Vachon GC, Ezike N, Brown-Walker M, et al. Improving access to diabetes care in an inner-city, community-based outpatient health center with a monthly open-access, multistation group visit program. *J Natl Med Assoc*. 2007;99(12):1327-36.

Vinci LM, Clark J, Buchholz N, et al. Improving diabetes care with nurse practitioner-led group visits and simple case management. *J Gen Intern Med*. 2006;21:72-72.

Watkinson M. Group visits improved concordance with American Diabetes Association practice guidelines in type 2 diabetes. *Evidence Based Nursing*. 2004;7(2):57-57.

Watts SA, Gee J, O'Day ME, et al. Nurse practitioner-led multidisciplinary teams to improve chronic illness care: The unique strengths of nurse practitioners applied to shared medical appointments/group visits. *J Am Acad Nurse Pract*. 2009;21(3):167-172.

Weber V, Bulger J, Sim J. Implementing a group visit model for adult patients with diabetes: A pilot. *J Gen Intern Med*. 2004;19:105-106.

Westheimer JM, Capello J, McCarthy C, et al. Employing a group medical intervention for hypertensive male veterans: an exploratory analysis. *Journal for Specialists in Group Work*. 2009;34(2):151-174.

Wheelock C, Savageau JA, Silk H, et al. Improving the health of diabetic patients through resident-initiated group visits. *Fam Med*. 2009;41(2):116-9.

Worth RC, Nicholson A, Bradley P. Shared care for diabetes in Chester: Preliminary experience with a 'clinic-wide' scheme. *Practical Diabetes*. 1990;7(6):266-268.

Yehle KS. A comparison of standard office visits and shared medical appointments in adults with heart failure. Touro University International; 2007.

Yehle KS, Sands LP, Rhynders PA, et al. The effect of shared medical visits on knowledge and self-care in patients with heart failure: a pilot study. *Heart Lung*. 2009;38(1):25-33.

Yu GC, Beresford R. Implementation of a chronic illness model for diabetes care in a family medicine residency program. *J Gen Intern Med*. 2010;25 Suppl 4:S615-9.

APPENDIX C. DATA ABSTRACTION ELEMENTS

Study Characteristics:
- Study Sites and Setting
- Study Design
- Comparator Type
- Enrollment Approach
- Study Enrollment/Study Completion (N's)
- Patient Eligibility Criteria for Study

Population Characteristics:
- Demographic
- Baseline Biophysical Characteristics

Intervention Components:
- Time period of intervention
- Type of model session and care team
- Number and duration of visits planned
- Number of health professionals present
- Was the prescribing clinician present?
- Size of patient group
- Were family members/friends invited to participate?
- Were medication changes made during the SMA visit?
- Did any clinician spend time with group members individually?
- Was the contact with the patients over the telephone outside of the SMA?
- Health professionals who conducted the educational session
- Theoretical orientation of the intervention
- Did group member have input on education topics?
- Topics covered during the session
- Strategy used with SMA group
- Were printed materials provided, and were they tailored?

Outcome Components:
- Target conditions
  - Biophysical markers postintervention values
    - HbA1c
    - Blood Pressures
    - Lipids
- Patient and staff experience
- Adherence (medication, visit, and self-management)
- Symptom severity
- Quality of life
- Functional status
- Resource utilization
- Direct cost and total cost
- Adverse effects

APPENDIX D. CRITERIA USED IN QUALITY ASSESSMENT

General Instructions:
For each risk of bias item, rate as "Yes," "No," or "Unclear." After considering each of the quality items, give the study an overall quality rating of good, fair, or poor.

Detailed Quality Items:
If an item is rated as "No," describe why in the comments column.

Randomization and allocation concealment:

a. *Randomization adequate?* Was the allocation sequence adequately generated?

❑ Yes   ❑ No   ❑ Not reported/Unclear

b. *Allocation concealment?* Was allocation adequately concealed?

❑ Yes   ❑ No   ❑ Not reported/Unclear

Outcomes:

a. *Outcome assessors blinded (hard outcomes)?* Were *Outcome assessors* blind to treatment assignment for "hard outcomes" such as mortality?

❑ Yes   ❑ No   ❑ Not reported/Unclear

b. *Outcome assessors blinded (soft outcomes)?* Were *Outcome assessors* blind to treatment assignment for "soft outcomes" such as symptoms?

❑ Yes   ❑ No   ❑ Not reported/Unclear

c. *Lack of measurement bias?* Were the measures used reliable and valid? If so, choose "Yes," indicating no important measurement bias.

❑ Yes   ❑ No   ❑ Not reported/Unclear

Data analysis:

a. *All outcomes reported?* Are reports of the study free of suggestion of selective outcome reporting (systematic differences between planned and reported findings)?

❑ Yes   ❑ No   ❑ Not reported/Unclear

b.   *Incomplete outcome data adequately addressed?*

❑ Yes (no systematic differences between groups in withdrawals from study and no high overall loss to follow-up; all eligible, randomized patients are included in analysis (ITT)

❑   No

❑   Not reported/Unclear

c.   *Adequate power for main effects?*

❑ Yes   ❑ No   ❑ Not reported/Unclear

Results:

a.   *Other selection bias?* Were systematic differences observed in baseline characteristics and and prognostic factors across the groups compared?

❑ Yes   ❑ No   ❑ Not reported/Unclear

b.   *Comparable groups maintained?* (Includes crossovers, adherence, and contamination). Consider issues of crossover (e.g., from one intervention to another), adherence (major differences in adherence to the interventions being compared), contamination (e.g., some members of control group get intervention), or other systematic differences in care that was provided.

❑ Yes   ❑ No   ❑ Not reported/Unclear

Conflict of interest:

a.   *Was there the absence of potential important conflict of interest?* The focus here is financial conflict of interest. If no financial conflict of interest (e.g., if funded by government or foundation and authors do not have financial relationships with drug/device manufacturer), then answer "Yes."

❑ Yes   ❑ No   ❑ Not reported/Unclear

* Items contained in Cochrane Risk of Bias Tool

<u>Overall study rating</u>:

Choose an item.

Please assign each study an overall quality rating of "Good," "Fair," or "Poor" based on the following definitions:

A "Good" study has the least bias, and results are considered valid. A good study has a clear description of the population, setting, interventions, and comparison groups; uses a valid approach to allocate patients to alternative treatments; has a low dropout rate; and uses appropriate means to prevent bias, measure outcomes, and analyze and report results.

A "Fair" study is susceptible to some bias but probably not enough to invalidate the results. The study may be missing information, making it difficult to assess limitations and potential problems. As the fair-quality category is broad, studies with this rating vary in their strengths and weaknesses. The results of some fair-quality studies are possibly valid, while others are probably valid.

A "Poor" rating indicates significant bias that may invalidate the results. These studies have serious errors in design, analysis, or reporting; have large amounts of missing information; or have discrepancies in reporting. The results of a poor-quality study are at least as likely to reflect flaws in the study design as to indicate true differences between the compared interventions.

Comments:

Form status:

❑ Fully complete – ready for export

❑ Not ready for export – should be discussed further/changes reconciled with the abstractor

APPENDIX E. PEER REVIEW COMMENTS

Reviewer	Comment	Response
Question 1: Are the objectives, scope, and methods for this review clearly described?		
1	Yes. The authors present the objectives and scope in a very succinct fashion. The methods are described in great detail. The key questions for review are very relevant in my opinion. Key question 1(KY 1) was well defined and the authors found 18 studies to evaluate. However KY2 and 3 are quite broad and not as clearly defined as KY 1. (Page 1, line 43, Page 2, Line 2). As there were not enough studies to address these questions, I can only speculate that if the questions were more focused, that the authors would have had better luck. They are to be commended for a thorough and detailed lit review, anyway to answer the call.	Thank you. The key questions were developed in collaboration with our stakeholders.
2	Yes. The terms "objectives" and "scope" were not used exactly; however the intent of this section was clearly described. The methods were superbly articulated.	Thank you.
3	Yes. Very clear.	Acknowledged
4	Yes. No comment.	Acknowledged
5	Yes. No comment.	Acknowledged
6	Yes. But comments under question 4.	Acknowledged
7	Yes. No comment.	Acknowledged
Question 2: Is there any indication of bias in our synthesis of the evidence?		
1	No. No comment.	Acknowledged
2	No. Risk of bias was evaluated when rating the body of evidence. Threats to internal validity of the systematic review conclusions were accounted for in potential selection bias, performance bias, and attribution and detection bias. Bias was accounted for by using criteria in the quality assessment tool in Appendix D for the review of the literature.	Thank you.
3	No. No comment.	Acknowledged
4	No. No comment.	Acknowledged
5	No. No comment.	Thank you.
6	No. But comments under question 4.	Acknowledged
7	No. No comment.	Acknowledged
Question 3: Are there any <u>published</u> or <u>unpublished</u> studies that we may have overlooked?		
1	No. Not that I am aware of.	Acknowledged
2	No. Not that I am aware of.	Acknowledged
3	No. No comment.	Acknowledged
4	No. I am not a SME on this topic so I may not be aware of some overlooked studies.	Acknowledged
5	Yes. I have unpublished retrospective pre-test/post-test study data awaiting consideration for publication from Diabetes Care Journal. N=1170 with ~ 1% A1c level drop.	Thank you for informing us about your data. We were unable to obtain a copy of this manuscript prior to finalizing our report.

Reviewer	Comment	Response
6	No. I am not aware of any, but I would be surprised if I knew of them from routine practice while the authors used a rigorous process. They do not include the many group interventions directed at weight control. I am not sure why these escaped their search criteria. I think they are not viewed as medical appointments by indexers, even though most would think the programs defined by the AHEAD study or even many MOVE! programs are medical encounters	Our focus on specific chronic conditions—asthma, coronary artery disease, congestive heart failure, chronic obstructive pulmonary disease, diabetes mellitus, hyperlipidemia, hypertension—was developed in collaboration with stakeholders. Obesity was considered but not included since medication management is not as prominent a component compared to the included conditions.
7	Yes. Published - Cohen, L. B., Taveira, T. H., Khatana, S. A., Dooley, A. G., Pirraglia, P. A., & Wu, W. C. (2011). Pharmacist-led shared medical appointments for multiple cardiovascular risk reduction in patients with type 2 diabetes. [Randomized Controlled Trial Research Support, Non-U.S. Gov't]. Diabetes Educ, 37(6), 801-812. doi: 10.1177/0145721711423980 Unpublished - Pharmacist-led Group Medical Visits to Help With Diabetes Management (MEDIC-1 year), NCT00554671	Thank you for making us aware of this study. It was published after our literature search but is now included in the review. Thank you for making us aware of this study. It has been added to the appendix of ongoing clinical trials.
	*Question 4: Please write additional suggestions or comments below. If applicable, please indicate the page and line numbers from the draft report*	
1	Few suggestions include: 1. (Page 3, Line 13) of executive summary: Mentioning the duration of the studies for the reader to get a snapshot would beneficial, as meaningful change in chronic disease takes time. See below. 2. (Page3, Line 37) of the executive summary: SMAs were associated with lower A1c than usual care (mean difference=0.58; 95% CI, -1.05 to -0.11) Again mentioning the time frame would be useful, especially as this was one of the main outcomes of their work. It is described on (page 22, line 18), assessed at 6 months to 4 years. 3. Page 24: Figure 4. Forest plots for meta-analysis on cholesterol. The headings for mean and SD says (mm Hg). Should say (mg/dl). I believe this is an error. 4. Page 24: Figure 5. Headings for mean SBP, should say (mmHg)	1. We added the range of followup to this section. 2. Thank you. This addition was made. 3. Thank you. This correction was made. 4. Thank you. This correction was made.

Reviewer	Comment	Response
1 cont.	I would like to commend the authors very highly for undertaking this extensive review. There is certainly great need to recognize, investigate and assess newer models of care for chronic illness in the 21st century. They present the current state of chronic illness care clearly, (page 8, line 22-26) which forms a nice background to the topic The methodology used is described in great detail and clear. Their conclusion after an extensive rigorous analysis of the literature highlights how complicated and inter-linked management of chronic disease really is. Their conclusion is not overstated.	Thank you.
	In the past decade, several breakthrough collaboratives introducing quality improvement methodology, rather than RCT's have been implemented in the US, mainly focusing on system improvements to address some of the key questions cited by the authors and addressing the six aims outlined by the Institute of medicine. This review did not analyze them. Only 18 studies qualified for analysis by the methods for SMA's being a newer model of care.	We followed the Cochrane Effective Practice and Organization of Care guidance, and included comparative patient or cluster RCTs, nonrandomized cluster controlled trials, controlled before-and-after studies, and interrupted time series designs. Any published breakthrough collaborative studies meeting these design specifications would have been included.
	As several components are inter-linked that leads to improvement in this model, it was hard to show significance with the rigor used in RCT's, the gold standard, as seen in this review. So in terms of future research, I am not convinced that large scale RCT's to address for e.g. diabetes outcomes will be feasible and answer the question described in (Table ES-2: evidence gaps and future research). One thought is to look at different models of care scientifically, to identify best practices and health systems with improved outcomes along with the economic cost for chronic illness management.	As stated above, we included comparative nonrandomized designs. We have modified the future research table to include these study design options.
	In conclusion, this paper has many strengths. (As cited by the authors). It is well described, clear and thoughtful with an exhaustive review and analysis of the literature. Going forward, it is an important topic for discussion in primary care and I greatly appreciate the opportunity to review this work.	Thank you.
2	On page 8 of the document (numbered as page 4), I noted in this paragraph, there needs to be a change in this word (see below in red). *Put page/paragraph here* *All three studies showed fewer hospital admissions in ......* In addition, on page 13 under the table where there are words describing what is meant by "provider", would you consider changing advance nurse practitioner to this Advanced Practice Registered Nurse (APRN) as this is the more correct term to describe the nurse provider. Thank you.	We have made this change. The typo "shower" was changed to "showed." We made the suggested change.
3	No comment from reviewer 5.	Acknowledged

Reviewer	Comment	Response
4	The scope of this data synthesis severely limited by limited number of high quality studies. It would seem that sufficient studies of sufficient design were not available to address KQ2 and KQ3. KQ1 of interest but only addresses initial questions of SMA effectiveness, and then only in diabetes. Some Tables not self-explanatory, such as Table ES-1 which refers to consistency, directness and precision but the definitions and measurement not clearly described.	We reviewed all Tables and edited or footnoted so that tables will "stand on their own."
	More analysis of issues raised in page 9 paragraph 2 would be helpful. Most of the SMA intervention studies suggest deployment of significant employee resources, sometimes on a limited number of patients in the group visit. These additional resources may have been largely responsible for the small improvement in intermediate outcomes seen in diabetes SMA. Left unresolved is whether it is worthwhile for facilities to invest these resources without clear return on investment. And for which patients?	We agree that this is a critical issue and attempted to determine factors associated with effect. Given the limits on intervention reporting and relatively small number of studies, our analysis did not identify the critical factors. For resource use, we were limited to the small amount of data reported.
5	p.9 2nd paragraph additional reasons for improved outcomes of SMA to consider-interprofessional synergism and motivational interviewing that goes on in the discussion section of SMA's.	Thank you. These are good points that have been added to the introduction.
	p.33 Table 6 Implementation issues-not clear that MD was most prevalent prescribing clinician if pharmacist & nurse practitioners listed with MD or without an MD were mentioned 11 studies and MD prescribers only as 8 times -may want to say have a prescribing clinician present.	We have attempted to clarify by describing the clinical leads and team composition in more detail (see KQ 3 results) and modifying the implementation table to reflect that a prescribing clinical is needed, rather than an MD.

Reviewer	Comment	Response
6	RE: EXECUTIVE SUMMARY I note that the executive summary is readable in length and well formatted. The writing is clear and crisp, which will be helpful to the eventual consumer.	Thank you.
	However, I am disappointed in several aspects of the presentation and data selected for presentations:	
	The Executive Summary emphasizes quantitative over qualitative commentary. There is very little discussion of the specific aspects of the interventions that are studied; if the reader is not familiar with what goes on in an SMA, then they won't know after reading this, either. Similarly, one has very little information about what the usual care control treatments are, or how one qualifies to get into the study. There is no exploration of the mechanism of action.	Thank you. We added a description of the common intervention components to the executive summary and the KQ 3 results. We have also added a section on the comparison condition in the initial description of the studies.
	Although I recognize that the summary must be brief, it is hard to imagine that all the tables pointing out that it is not possible to draw definitive conclusions based on a couple of studies of non-diabetic high users, or draw conclusions about economic effects when most studies did not report them.	Results are briefly summarized in text. The table also summarizes results but adds the strength of evidence (SOE). Unfortunately, the SOE was insufficient for many outcomes
	This is especially disappointing since the readers are not naïve – they are likely to be aware of the literature suggesting a benefit from SMA based on prominent studies, several in VA, that have had this finding. What the reader needs is guidance regarding what one should or should not do if one is attempting to be evidence based. I think that requires description of commonalities in the study designs, even if you can't comment on whether one aspect or another was demonstrably better.	Unfortunately, the literature does not yet establish the characteristics of SMA associated with benefit. However, in the KQ 3 results, we describe the common features and echo these findings in the discussion.
	Since the introduction suggests a couple mechanisms of action, perhaps one could say whether the results say anything about these. In the case of improved access, for example, I guess the answer is that this is NOT the mechanism, since the control people would have also benefited from the provider having more clinic slots. Similarly, if the mechanism were expertise, I would like to see commentary on the expertise of the providers who participated in the SMA – my sense from the articles I have reviewed is that they are not content area experts.	Thank you. This is a good point, but few studies reported intermediate outcomes (e.g., self-management behaviors) or provider training. We report the available results and have added to the discussion the point that few studies report on the potential mechanisms of action.

Reviewer	Comment	Response
6 cont.	RE: METHODS I think that these are well described. But I wish that there was more of a sense that clinical experts were doing the synthesis and they were thinking about how they made sense. The AHRQ methodology does not seem to exclude this. Moreover, I acknowledge it seems like it is not very rigorous and might be open to bias on the part of the reviewers. So I think that this is why you have people like me review the opinion and offer a counterpoint. And I am confident that the Durham VA and Duke has a lot of people who could offer opinions and give the consumer confidence that the recommendations are in the end based on opinion, but very well informed and vetted opinion.	The research team included physicians (one who is expert in shared medical appointments) and psychologists. Our goal was to summarize the evidence so that policy makers could incorporate the best available evidence into decision making.
	Thus, I would like to see an attempt to present the rationale for why they think they won't change their mind (i.e., strength of evidence "High") or that they are not yet convinced. I would not want this to be devoid of quantitative thinking, rather, I would like an exposition of why they think what they think – this can be that it just does not make sense or that it is very consistent with lots of less strong studies or that the quantitative analysis is particularly convincing or is subject to error due to some methodological consideration, despite a nominally significant p value or important effect size (e.g., the condemnation of IMG carotid endarterectomy complication rates based on a trivial number of cases – Ann Intern Med 1990;113:747-753).	The approach to assigning SOE is summarized in the methods section. The summary table in the discussion presents our judgments about each domain (study design, risk of bias, consistency, directness, precision) that forms the foundation for these judgments.
	RE: RESULTS: I am surprised that there is no description of the eligibility criterion. Obviously, the DM trials required the patients to have DM, but there is no information about whether this was to be poorly controlled or of a certain duration, or if the patients had to have a stable medical regimen or be taking or not taking insulin or ??	Thank you. We have added descriptions of the eligibility criteria to the results (see KQ 1).
	Outcomes are well reported in tabular form. Although there are no statistically effects by study or patient characteristics, I would have liked some exploration of individual examples with greater or smaller effect size, and some assessment of why one had more effect than another.	Effects were consistent for blood pressure outcomes but varied for glucose control and HRQOL. We explored three factors hypothesized a priori to be related to effect size: baseline severity, intervention robustness, and study quality.

Reviewer	Comment	Response
6 cont.	It is presumably because the study authors did not include the information, but one wonders if there are any process measures like medication changes or behavior changes that could explain the change in control. For example, with all the BP improvement, did this reflect a drop in weight, a change in prescribed medication, a change in medication adherence, a change in physical activity or what ? Or do we just not know? It seems most likely that this reflects a medication effect, since the effect on A1c, LDL and BP are all sensitive to this, and there is no evidence of a change in weight – I assume this was examined and will be reported in the revised version.	The authors of the individual studies did not provide this data consistently. A few studies report effects on self-management behaviors and these results are reported in KQ 1 "treatment experience and adherence outcomes." We also abstracted information on medication changes and report these results in the same section
	RE: DISCUSSION: I love that there is an explicit paragraph labeled "Should SMAs be Implemented?" But I am disappointed that it does not appear that they answer this question. Since the VA in particular paid for this synthesis, one would think there would at least be an answer for VA. It might be something along the lines of "The evidence available suggests that the VA should be implementing an SMA in all hospitals. This should be made available for all patients who have inadequate control. However, one should require referral by the primary care provider." One would obviously provide caveats and nuance the presentation, but it is unfortunate that when the explicit goal is to help policy makers change policy, the guidance is vague.	Our goal is to synthesize the evidence to inform policymaking. Although we try to describe some of the considerations (in addition to evidence of intervention effect) that might influence policy, it is not our role to prescribe policy.
	RE: APPENDIX C – DATA ELEMENTS ABSTRACTED Hard to imagine that weight was not abstracted from at least some of the studies, given that all the disease specific studies were about diabetes.	Weight was not specified as an outcome of interest by our study team or stakeholders.
	"Health professionals who conducted the educational session" is not reported with much specificity – that is, we see only MD as the descriptor. Is there evidence of specialists versus generalists? The same question applies to the pharmacists. Or are they just people who are interested in the area or researcher team members.	Specialty, training and experience of the MD professionals were almost never described.
	RE: APPENDIX G – Study characteristics of included studies The column labeled "Target condition HBA1c % (for total population)" appears to be mislabeled. The number in parentheses seems to be the standard deviation, not the value of A1c for the total population. Or the percent of the total population included – I am not sure what they mean by this.	Thank you. We relabeled the column to improve clarity.
	Usual care could have been described in more detail. Particularly in situations where the DM control was poor at baseline, one would imagine that the correct comparator would be some other, non-group approach to improved control – probably as simple as having the prescribing provider see the person for better control.	We have added a paragraph describing the Comparison Conditions in more detail in the "Study Characteristics" section of the results.
	Since the introduction suggests that access to an expert provider might be the mechanism of action, I wonder if there is information about the training of the MD or pharmacist.	Unfortunately, information about the specialty training and experience of the MD clinician or clinical pharmacist was give rarely.

Reviewer	Comment	Response
7	Other elements to assess in explaining heterogeneity of study results in diabetes is the clinician expertise in diabetes and group management, e.g. do the clinician(s) have training in diabetes or conduction of group visits prior to starting the trial – such as being a certified diabetes educator, do the clinician(s) manage diabetes in other settings – such as individual diabetes clinics, how many disciplines were in the team, etc.	Although this is a good idea, and could explain heterogeneity in intervention effects, clinician expertise and certification as a diabetes educator were not described consistently enough for analysis.
	**Optional Dissemination and Implementation Questions**	
	*Question 5: Are there any VA clinical performance measures, programs, quality improvement measures, patient care services, or conferences that will be directly affected by this report? If so, please provide detail.*	
1	I do not work in the VA setting, so am unable to comment on this.	Acknowledged
2	The Office of Nursing Service (ONS) conducts courses on EBP; use of this document may enhance learning for the participants who would attend this conference; given that the EBP course is for the properly targeted audience. The other group that could benefit is the Clinical Practice Portfolio of the ONS as this ES is timely to impact recommendations for intervention for both PACT and Specialty Care services. In addition, a presentation on the findings would be beneficial for the Advanced Practice Nursing Advisory Group as this group of providers would be influenced by these findings.	Acknowledged Acknowledged
3	PACT compass, Office of Patient Care Service, Office of Nursing Service, Office of Academic Affiliations: Centers of Excellence in Primary Care Education	Acknowledged
4	PACT implementation included an emphasis on SMA and group visits as a means to enhance access and implement a chronic care model. The ability to improve access is not addressed by this data synthesis. A SMA of reasonable size might improve access by reducing reliance on routine clinic visits. This hypothesis was not evaluated. A concern from the perspective of PACT is that the SMA might adversely affect patient continuity with their primary care provider. The information regarding whether the intervention preserved patient continuity with the provider or not is not provided. An evaluation of the benefits of SMA versus the trade-offs might ultimately be very helpful.	Acknowledged Most studies describe the intervention as additional care, rather than a substitute for primary care. We have added a statement to this effect in the discussion. No studies reported access outcomes directly or information on continuity with their PCP. Few reported effects on patient experience.
5	PACT initiative in Primary Care is promoting SMA's.	Acknowledged
6	The authors are clear that there is not enough evidence that we can say that use or non-use of SMA is a quality issue. I think there are a number of conferences where the results will be of interest – certainly HSR and QUERI and hopefully the leadership meetings.	The results of this review and a parallel "realist" review are being presented at the July 2012 HSR&D conference.
7	PACT compass that includes SMA as one of its components, in addition to the traditional diabetes performance measures in Primary care	Acknowledged

Reviewer	Comment	Response
Question 6: Please provide any recommendations on how this report can be revised to more directly address or assist implementation needs.		
1	No comments by reviewer 2	
2	Report is very well done. Are companion presentations done in conjunction with the report (PowerPoint, to be used for presenting to interested groups)?	Thank you. There will be a presentation at the July 2012 HSR&D/QUERI meeting.
3	Executive summary very direct and to the point. Recommendations for future research offer usable directions	Thank you.
4	More information about the intervention would have been helpful. Key elements that may result in successful implementation are hinted at in Table 6, but are not fully discussed. This table is also not self-explanatory: for example what is meant by "Team continuity"?	We revised Table 6 and footnoted other tables to more improve clarity. Detailed information on the intervention is presented in Appendix H and summarized in Table 3.
5	A table of the roles of each providers (along with quality) in the studies would help as sites try to implement SMA's	Although team composition was described, roles of individual providers were not described consistently enough to develop the requested table.
6	See response to #4	Addressed above.
7	I believe this report is an unbiased assessment and synthesis of current literature and clearly points out the strengths and weaknesses of the available data	Thank you.
Question 7: Please provide us with contact details of any additional individuals/stakeholders who should be made aware of this report.		
1	No. No comment	Acknowledged
2	Once completed: Christine Engstrom, Anna Alt-White	Acknowledged
3	PACT e-mail group, Centers of Excellence in Primary Care Education	Acknowledged
4	Richard Stark; Joanne Shear	Acknowledged
5	No comment	Acknowledged
6	None in particular	Acknowledged
7	No comment	Acknowledged

APPENDIX F. ONGOING CLINICAL TRIALS

Table F-1. Ongoing clinical trials

Official study title	Organization	Intervention	Comparator	Sponsor and ClinicalTrials.gov ID	Funding Start/Stop	Status
Interprofessional Training for Improving Diabetes Care	Government	Shared medical appointments to promote establishing collaborative teams (ReSPECT)	Traditional diabetes education and teleconsultation	Department of Veterans Affairs NCT00854594	Sep 2010–Sep 2012	Recruiting
Initiating Diabetic Group Visits in Newly Diagnosed Diabetics in an Urban Academic Medical Practice	University-affiliated clinic	Group Visit	Standard individual medical appointment	Oregon Health and Science University NCT01497301	Feb 2012–Feb 2013	Not yet open for participation
Heart Failure Group Clinic Appointments: Rehospitalization	University-affiliated clinic	Heart Failure Group Clinic Appointments	Standard heart failure education	Carol Smith, RN, PhD, FAAN (NHLBI) NCT00439842	Mar 2007–Sep 2012	Ongoing, but not recruiting
Group Intervention for DM Guideline Implementation	Government	Pharmacist-led group medical visits for patients with type 2 diabetes mellitus	Usual care	Department of Veterans Affairs NCT00554671	May 2008–June 2012	Ongoing, but not recruiting participants

Abbreviations: DM=diabetes mellitus; NHLBI=National Heart, Lung, and Blood Institute

APPENDIX G. SMA STUDY CHARACTERISTICS

Table G-1. SMA study characteristics

Study	Location Setting Organization Total N	Age in Years (SD) Sex (%) Race/ethnicity (%)	Target Condition Mean Baseline HBA1c % (SD) (for Diabetes Studies)	SMA Planned Visits Study Duration	Comparator	Quality
Beck, 1997	US Primary care HMO 321	73.5 (NR) Male (34%) NR	Chronically ill older adults Not applicable	12 >12 months	Usual care	Poor
Bray, 2005	US Primary care University-affiliated clinic 160	59.4 (14.3) Male (44%) NR	Diabetes; hypertension HBA1c: 8.2 (2.4)	4 12 months	Usual care	Fair
Clancy, 2003	US Primary care University-affiliated clinic 120	54.0 (NR) Male (22%) Black (77.5%)	Type 2 diabetes HBA1c: 10.4 (NR)	6 6 months	Usual care	Good
Clancy , 2007	US Primary care University-affiliated clinic 186	56.0 (NR) Male (28%) Black (83.3%)	Type 2 diabetes HBA1c: 9.1 (2.0)	12 12 months	Usual care	Fair
Cohen, 2011	US Primary care VA Health system 99	69.8 (10.7) Male (100%) NR	Type 2 diabetes HbA1c: 7.8 (1.0)	4 once weekly + 5 monthly booster session 6 months	Usual care	Fair
Culhane-Pera, 2005	US Federally qualified health center Government 61	56.8 (NR) Male (36%) NR	Type 2 diabetes HBA1c: 9.4 (NR)	7 visits 28 months	Usual care	Poor
Edelman, 2010	US Primary care VA Health system 239	62.0 (9.7) Male (96%) Black (59.0%)	Diabetes; hypertension HBA1c: 9.2 (1.4)	7 visits 12 months	Usual care	Good
Gutierrez, 2011	US Primary care University-affiliated clinic 103	NR (NR) Male (NR) Hispanic (100%)	Type 2 diabetes HBA1c: NR (NR)	36 visits offered 17 months	Usual care	Poor

Study	Location Setting Organization Total N	Age in Years (SD) Sex (%) Race/ethnicity (%)	Target Condition Mean Baseline HBA1c % (SD) (for Diabetes Studies)	SMA Planned Visits Study Duration	Comparator	Quality
Kirsh, 2007	US Primary care VA Health system 79	61.0 (9.9) Male (NR) NR	Type 2 diabetes HBA1c: 10.1 (NR)	NA (drop-in) 4 months)	Usual care	Fair
Levine, 2010	US Primary care HMO 1236	78.2 (7.2) Male (35%) NR	High usage of clinic services Not applicable	12 visits 12 months	Usual care	Fair
Naik, 2011	US Primary care VA Health system 87	63.6 (7.9) Male (NR) Black (31.0%)	Type 2 diabetes HBA1c: 8.8 (1.3)	4 visits 3 months intervention; 12 months followup	Enhanced usual care (2 required diabetes group education sessions)	Good
Sadur, 1999	US Primary care HMO 185	56.0 (9.1) Male (57%) White (74.6%)	Types 1 and 2 diabetes HBA1c: 9.7 (1.7)	6 visits 6 months	Usual care	Good
Scott, 2004	US Primary care HMO 294	74.1 (7.5) Male (41%) NR	Older; high usage of clinic services Not applicable	24 visits 24 months	Usual care	Fair
Taveira, 2010	US Primary care VA Health system 118	64.4 (10.3) Male (95%) White (91.0%)	Type 2 diabetes HBA1c: 8.0 (1.3)	4 visits 1 month (outcomes reported at 4 months)	Usual care	Fair
Taveira, 2011	US Primary care VA Health system 88	60.8 (9.6) Male (98%) White (99%)	Types 1 and 2 diabetes HBA1c: 8.4 (1.8)	9 visits 6 months	Usual care	Good
Trento, 2001	Italy Diabetes clinic University-affiliated clinic 112	61.5 (NR) Male (54%) NR	Type 2 diabetes HBA1c: 7.4 (1.4)	7-8 visits 24 months	Usual care plus individual education sessions	Fair
Trento, 2005	Italy Diabetes clinic University-affiliated clinic 62	Median 27-31 (NR) Male (60%) NR	Type 1 diabetes HBA1c: 8.7 (1.2)	15 visits 36 months	Usual care plus individual education sessions	Fair

Shared Medical Appointments for Chronic Medical Conditions

Study	Location Setting Organization Total N	Age in Years (SD) Sex (%) Race/ethnicity (%)	Target Condition Mean Baseline HBA1c % (SD) (for Diabetes Studies)	SMA Planned Visits Study Duration	Comparator	Quality
Trento, 2010	Italy Diabetes clinic University-affiliated clinic 815	69.3 (8.4) Male (51%) NR	Type 2 diabetes HBA1c: 7.8 (1.6)	14 visits 48 months	Usual care; followup scheduled every 3 months	Good
Wagner, 2001	US Primary care HMO 707	60.7(NR) Male (53%) White (72.8%)	Types 1 and 2 diabetes HBA1c: 7.5 (NR)	8 visits 24 months	Usual care	Fair

APPENDIX H. SMA INTERVENTION COMPONENTS

Table H-1. SMA interventions: team and process components

Study	Clinical Team			Group				Group Visit Processes		
	Clinical disciplines	Team continuity	Team size	Closed?	Group size	Family or peers allowed?	Individual breakouts?	Medication changes?	Visit duration (minutes)	Telephone contacts?
Beck, 1997	MD, RN, and psychologists (as guest lecturers)	Specific group but rotated	≥2	Yes	8[a]	Yes	Yes	Yes	120	Yes
Bray, 2005	MD, RN, and/or others (type NR)	Yes	2	Yes	3-12	NR	Yes	Yes	120	NR
Clancy, 2003	MD, nurse practitioner, and guest presenters	Yes	2-3	Yes	19-20	NR	Yes	Yes	120	No
Clancy, 2007	MD and RN	Yes	2	Yes	6-7	No	Yes	Yes	120	No
Cohen, 2011	Pharmacist, RN, physical therapist and dietitian	Yes	4	Yes	4-6	Yes	NR	Yes	60	No
Culhane-Pera, 2005	Exercise specialist, MD, RN, and social worker	Yes	7	Yes	10-16	Yes	NR	Yes	210	NR
Edelman, 2010	Health educator, MD, pharmacist, or RN	Yes	3	Yes	7-8	No	Yes	Yes	90-120	Yes
Gutierrez, 2011	MD, pharmacist, RN, and social worker	NR	7	No	NR	NR	NR	NR[b]	NR	NR
Kirsh, 2007	MD, nurse practitioner, pharmacist, psychologist, and/or RN	Yes	5	No	≤8	NR	Yes	Yes	Varied	NR
Levine, 2010	MD and nurse practitioner	Yes	3	Yes	25	NR	Yes	Yes	>60 / 90	NR / NR/unclear
Naik, 2011	MD	Yes	≥2	Yes	5-7	No	Yes	Yes	120	No

Shared Medical Appointments for Chronic Medical Conditions

| Study | Clinical Team | | Group | | Group Visit Processes | | | |
	Clinical disciplines	Team continuity / Team size	Closed? / Group size	Family or peers allowed?	Individual breakouts?	Medication changes?	Visit duration (minutes)	Telephone contacts?
Sadur, 1999	Behaviorist, dietician, pharmacist, and RN	Yes / 4	Yes / 10-18	No	Yes	Yes	120	Yes
Scott, 2004	MD, pharmacist, RN, physical therapist, and occupational therapist	Yes / ≥2	No / 7.7[a]	Yes	Yes	Yes	120	No
Taveira, 2010	Dietician, pharmacist, physical therapist, and RN	Yes / Unclear	Yes / 4-8	Yes	NR	Yes	120	No
Taveira, 2011	Pharmacist and RN	Yes / Unclear	No / 4-6	Yes	No	Yes	120	No
Trento, 2001	Health educator and MD	Partial[c] / 2-3	Yes / 9-10	Yes	Yes	Yes	50-80	No
Trento, 2005	MD and psychopedagogist	Partial[c] / 2	Yes / 6-7	Yes	Yes	Yes	40-80	No
Trento, 2010	Health educator and MD	Partial[c] / 2	Yes / 9-10	Yes	Yes	Yes	60	No
Wagner, 2001	MD, pharmacist, and RN	Yes / 3	Yes / 6-10	NR	Yes	NR	60	No

[a]Group size: In these cases, a mean value rather than a range is reported in the article.

[b]Medication changes: This article did not clearly report whether medication changes were made as part of the group process; however, it is implied in that an MD and a pharmacist were usually present, and the intervention group both lowered their HbA1c and started taking more aspirin than the control group.

[c]Trento studies: The investigators relied on a pool of health providers for group intervention, which may provide patients with the possibility to see the same provider more than once—hence, team continuity is partially present.

Shared Medical Appointments for Chronic Medical Conditions

Table H-2: SMA interventions: educational and behavioral components

Study	Leader(s) of Educational Session	Behavioral Approach	Patients Input on Topics?	Topics	Behavioral Strategies	Print Material?
Beck, 1997	MD, pharmacist, RN, or other team member	NR	No	Medication management, nutrition, physical activity	NR	Yes, generic
Bray, 2005	RN or other team member	NR	NR	Disease-specific education, medication management, nutrition	Goal-setting, personalized plan	NR
Clancy, 2003	MD, RN, or guest lecturers	NR	Yes	Disease-specific education, medication management, nutrition, physical activity	NR	NR
Clancy , 2007	MD	NR	Yes	Disease-specific education, medication management, nutrition, physical activity	NR	NR
Cohen, 2011	Pharmacist	NR	No	Disease specific education, medication management, nutrition, physical activity	Goal-setting, homework assignments, personalized care plan, self-monitoring	Yes
Culhane-Pera, 2005	RN	NR	No	Disease-specific education, medication management, nutrition, physical activity	Goal-setting, problem-solving skills	NR
Edelman, 2005	Health educator or RN	NR	Yes	Disease-specific education, medication management, nutrition, physical activity	Personalized care plan	Yes, generic
Gutierrez, 2011	Social worker	NR	NR	NR	NR	NR
Kirsh, 2007	Health psychologist	NR	NR	Disease-specific education nutrition, smoking cessation	Personalized plan	Yes, generic
Levine, 2010	MD or RN	NR	Yes	Medication management, nutrition, physical activity	NR	Yes, generic
Naik, 2011	Study clinician	NR	No	Disease-specific education, medication management	Goal-setting, personalized plan, problem-solving skills, self- monitoring	Yes, tailored
Sadur, 1999	Dietician, health behavior specialist, pharmacist, podiatrist, or RN	NR	Yes	Disease-specific education, physical activity	Personalized plan	NR
Scott, 2004	Dietician, MD, pharmacist, physical therapist, or RN	NR	Yes	Disease-specific education, medication management, nutrition, physical activity	NR	Yes tailored
Taveira, 2010	Dietician, pharmacist, physical therapist, or RN	Stages of change	No	Disease-specific education, medication management, nutrition, physical activity, smoking cessation	NR	Yes, tailored

Study	Leader(s) of Educational Session	Behavioral Approach	Patients Input on Topics?	Topics	Behavioral Strategies	Print Material?
Taveira, 2011	Nutritionist, pharmacist, or RN	Stages of change	No	Disease-specific education, medication management, nutrition, physical activity, smoking cessation	NR	Yes, tailored
Trento, 2001	MD or health educator	Patient-centered adult learning	No	Disease-specific education, medication management, nutrition, physical activity, smoking cessation	Homework assignment, problem-solving skills, self-monitoring	Yes, tailored
Trento, 2005	MD or health educator	Patient-centered adult learning	Yes	Disease-specific education, medication management, nutrition, physical activity, self-care	Homework assignment, problem-solving skills, self-monitoring	Yes, tailored
Trento, 2010	MD or health educator	Patient-centered adult learning	No	Disease-specific education, medication management, nutrition, physical activity, smoking cessation	Homework assignment, problem-solving skills, self-monitoring	Yes, tailored
Wagner, 2001	RN or other health professional	NR	No	Disease-specific education	Self-monitoring	Yes, generic

APPENDIX I. GLOSSARY

Abstract screening

The stage in a systematic review during which titles and abstracts of articles identified in the literature search are screened for inclusion or exclusion based on established criteria. Articles that pass the abstract screening stage are promoted to the full-text review stage.

Allocation concealment

The method by which randomization assignment is concealed from participants and investigators before and during the enrollment process. Common processes are central allocation (telephone or web-based, pharmacy or off-site statistician controlled randomization sequence generation and sequentially numbered, opaque, sealed envelopes. Allocation concealment concentrates on preventing selection and confounding biases, safeguards the assignment sequence *before and until* allocation, and can always be successfully implemented

Area under the curve (AUC)

The area under the receiver operating characteristic (ROC) curve. The summary receiver operator characteristic (SROC) curve and the AUC have been proposed as a way to assess diagnostic data in the context of a meta-analysis. The accuracy of a diagnostic test depends on how well the test separates the group being tested into those with and without the condition in question.

Case-control study

A retrospective, analytical, observational study often based on secondary data in which the proportion of cases with a potential risk factor are compared to the proportion of controls (individuals without the disease or condition) with the same risk factor. The common association measure for a case-control study is the odds ratio. These studies are commonly used for initial, inexpensive evaluation of risk factors and are particularly useful for rare conditions or for risk factors with long induction periods. Unfortunately, due to the potential for many forms of bias in this study type, case control studies provide relatively weak empirical evidence even when properly executed.

Case report

A description of a single case, typically describing the manifestations, clinical course, and prognosis of that case. Due to the wide range of natural biologic variability in these aspects, a single case report provides little empirical evidence to the clinician. A case report does describe how others diagnosed and treated the condition and what the clinical outcome was.

Case series

A descriptive, observational study of a series of cases, typically describing the manifestations, clinical course, and prognosis of a condition. A case series provides weak empirical evidence because of the lack of comparability unless the findings are dramatically different from expectations. Case series are best used as a source of hypotheses for investigation by stronger study designs, leading some to suggest that the case series should be regarded as clinicians talking to researchers. Unfortunately, the case series is the most common study type in the clinical literature.

ClinicalTrials.gov

A registry and results database of federally and privately supported clinical trials conducted in the United States and around the world. ClinicalTrials.gov provides information about a trial's purpose, location, participant characteristics, among other details.

Cochrane Database of Systematic Reviews

A bibliographic database of peer-reviewed systematic reviews and protocols prepared by the Cochrane Review Groups in The Cochrane Collaboration.

Cochran's Q test

A nonparametric statistic to test for differences in intervention effects between studies. Because the test statistic is often underpowered, the threshold for statistically significant differences in intervention effects is often set at $p<0.10$.

Cohort study

A prospective, analytical, observational study based on data, usually primary, from a followup period of a group in which some have had, have, or will have the exposure of interest, to determine the association between that exposure and an outcome. Cohort studies are susceptible to bias by differential loss to followup, the lack of control over risk assignment, and the potential for zero time bias when the cohort is assembled. Because of their prospective nature, cohort studies are stronger than case-control studies when well executed, but they also are more expensive. Because of their observational nature, cohort studies do not provide empirical evidence that is as strong as that provided by properly executed randomized controlled clinical trials.

Companion article

A publication from a trial that is not the article containing the main results of that trial. It may be a methods paper, a report of subgroup analyses, a report of combined analyses, or other auxiliary topic that adds information to the interpretation of the main publication.

Confidence interval (CI)

The range in which a particular result (such as a laboratory test) is likely to occur for everyone in the population of interest a specified percentage of the time known as the confidence level or confidence coefficient. It is an interval calculated from a study's observations used to estimate the reliability of the estimate of a parameter. The most common confidence level is 95%. For example, a confidence interval with a 95% confidence level is intended to give the assurance that, if the statistical model is correct, then taken over all the data that *might* have been obtained, the true value of the parameter will be found within the given interval 95% of the time.

Consistency

Extent to which effect size and direction vary within and across studies; inconsistency may be due to heterogeneity across PICOTS.

Cumulative Index to Nursing and Allied Health Literature (CINAHL)

A collection of medical databases of nursing and allied health literature.

Data abstraction

The stage of a systematic review that involves a pair of trained researchers extracting reported findings specific to the research questions from the full-text articles that met the established inclusion criteria. These data form the basis of the evidence synthesis.

Directness

Degree to which outcomes that are important to users of the comparative effectiveness review (patients, clinicians, or policymakers) are encompassed by trial data.

Embase

A database containing bibliographic records with citations, abstracts, and indexing derived from biomedical and pharmacological articles in peer-reviewed journals.

Exclusion criteria

The criteria, or standards, set out before a study or review. Exclusion criteria are used to determine whether a person should participate in a research study or whether an individual study should be excluded in a systematic review. Exclusion criteria may include age, previous treatments, and other medical conditions.

External validity

The extent to which clinical research studies apply to broader populations. A research study has external validity if its results can be generalized to the larger population.

Forest plot

A visual display of information from individual studies in a meta-analysis. A forest plot shows the amount of variation between the results of the studies as well as an estimate of the overall result of all the studies together. A horizontal line represents the 95% confidence interval (CI) of the "effect" observed in the studies.

Full-text review

The stage of a systematic review in which a pair of trained researches evaluates the full-text of study articles for potential inclusion in the review.

GRADE

Grading of Recommendations Assessment, Development and Evaluation (GRADE), a systematic approach to evaluating the overall body of research evidence and rating the quality of medical evidence and the strength of clinical recommendations.

Health-related quality of life (HRQOL)

Aspects of overall quality of life that can be clearly shown to affect health—either physical or mental health.

I^2

A statistic that describes the percentage (range from 0-100%) of total variation across studies due to heterogeneity between study characteristics rather than due to chance. Heterogeneity is categorized as low, moderate or high based on I^2 values of 25, 50 or 75%, respectively. It is considered an indication of consistency or inconsistency across studies in a meta-analysis.

Inclusion criteria

The criteria, or standards, set out before the systematic review. Inclusion criteria are used to determine whether an individual study can be included in a systematic review. Inclusion criteria may include population, study design, gender, age, type of disease being treated, previous treatments, and other medical conditions.

Intent-to-treat analysis

A method of analyzing results of a randomized controlled trial that includes in the analysis all cases that should have received a treatment regimen but for some reason did not. All cases allocated to each arm of the trial are analyzed together as representing that treatment arm, regardless of whether they received or completed the prescribed regimen.

Interquartile range (IQR)

A measure of the spread of or dispersion within a data set. The IQR is the width of an interval that contains the middle 50 percent of the sample, so it is smaller than the range and its value is less affected by outliers.

Meta-analysis

A way of combining data from many different research studies. A meta-analysis is a statistical process that combines the findings from individual studies.

Meta-regression analyses

An extension of meta-analysis to subgroups that allows the effect of continuous, as well as categorical, characteristics to be investigated if sufficient studies examining the same characteristics may be compared. In principle, it allows the effect of multiple factors to be investigated simultaneously. In meta-regression, the outcome variable is the effect estimate (e.g., a mean difference, etc.). The explanatory variables are characteristics of studies that might influence the size of the intervention effect.

Mixed effects

Statistical models that include both fixed (nonrandom) and random effects.

National Committee for Quality Assurance (NCQA)

A nonprofit organization dedicated to improving health care quality.

National Quality Forum (NQF)

A nonprofit organization that promotes change through development and implementation of a national strategy for health care quality measurement and reporting.

Negative predictive value (NPV)

The likelihood that people with a negative test result would not have a condition. The higher the value of the negative predictive value (for example, 99 percent would usually be considered a high value), the more useful the test is for predicting that people do not have the condition.

Nonrandomized study

Any quantitative study estimating the effectiveness of an intervention (harm or benefit) that does not use randomization to allocate units to comparison groups (including studies where "allocation" occurs in the course of usual treatment decisions or peoples' choices; i.e., studies usually called "observational"). There are many possible types of nonrandomized intervention studies, including cohort studies, case-control studies, controlled before-and-after studies, interrupted-time-series studies, and controlled trials that do not use appropriate randomization strategies (sometimes called quasi-randomized studies).

Observational study

A study in which the investigators do not seek to intervene but simply observe the course of events. Changes or differences in one characteristic (e.g., whether or not people received the intervention of interest) are studied in relation to changes or differences in other characteristics (e.g., whether or not they died), without action by the investigator. Observational studies provide weaker empirical evidence than do experimental studies because of the potential for large confounding biases to be present when there is an unknown association between a factor and an outcome.

Odds ratio

A ratio of the odds of having the outcome of interest in a group with a particular exposure, symptom, or characteristic of interest, to the odds of outcome in a group that does not have the exposure/symptom/characteristic. An odds ratio of 1 indicates that the outcome is equally likely to occur in both groups. An odds ratio of 4 indicates that the outcome is 4 times more likely to be present in the group that has the symptom or characteristic of interest, compared with the group that does not have this symptom. When outcomes are infrequent, the odds ratio is a good approximation of the risk ratio.

Outlier

An observation in a data set that is far removed in value from the others in the data set. It is an unusually large or an unusually small value compared to the others.

Patient-centered adult learning

An approach used in the professional–patient interaction. Common elements are empathic communication, acknowledgement, realistic expectations, goal negotiation, guided problem-solving, individualized strategies, and ongoing support.

PICOTS

Population, intervention, comparator, outcome, timing, setting.

Positive predictive value (PPV)

Indicates the likelihood that a person with a positive test result would actually have the condition for which the test is used. The higher the value of the positive predictive value (for example, 90 percent would be considered a high value), the more useful the test is for predicting that the person has the condition.

Precision

The degree of certainty for estimate of effect with respect to a specific outcome.

Preferred Reporting Items of Systematic Reviews and Meta-Analyses (PRISMA)

An evidence-based minimum set of items for reporting in systematic reviews and meta-analyses.

Probability

The likelihood (or chance) that an event will occur. In a clinical research study, it is the number of times a condition or event occurs in a study group divided by the number of people being studied.

Process of care or performance measure

Quality measures used to gauge how well an entity provides care to its patients. Measures are based on scientific evidence and usually reflected in guidelines, standards of care or practice parameters.

Prospective observational study

A clinical research study in which people who presently have a certain condition or receive a particular treatment are followed over time and compared with another group of people who are not affected by the condition.

PsycINFO

An abstracting and indexing database of peer-reviewed literature in the behavioral sciences and mental health.

Publication bias

The tendency of researchers to publish experimental findings that have a positive result, while not publishing the findings when the results are negative or inconclusive. The effect of publication bias is that published studies may be misleading. When information that differs from that of the published study is not known, people are able to draw conclusions using only information from the published studies.

PubMed

A database of citations for biomedical literature from MEDLINE, life science journals, and online books in the fields of medicine, nursing, dentistry, veterinary medicine, the health care system, and preclinical sciences.

QUADAS

Quality Assessment of the Diagnostic Accuracy Studies, a tool that uses a standard methodology to judge the quality of individual studies in a systematic review.

Quasi-experimental study

A quasi-experimental study manipulates a variable between two or more groups, but participants are not randomly assigned to groups. Quasi-experimental study designs, such as nonrandomized pre-post studies, are frequently used when it is not logistically feasible or ethical to conduct a randomized controlled trial.

Quasi-random allocation

Methods of allocating people to a trial that are not random but were intended to produce similar groups when used to allocate participants. Quasi-random methods include allocation by the person's date of birth, by the day of the week or month of the year, by a person's medical record number, or just allocating every alternate person. In practice, these methods of allocation are relatively easy to manipulate, introducing selection bias.

Randomized controlled trial

A prospective, analytical, experimental study using primary data generated in the clinical environment. Individuals similar at the beginning of the trial are randomly allocated to two or more treatment groups and the outcomes the groups are compared after sufficient followup time. Properly executed, the RCT is the strongest evidence of the clinical efficacy of preventive and therapeutic procedures in the clinical setting.

Relative risk (RR)

A comparison of the risk of a particular event for different groups of people. Relative risk is usually used to estimate exposure to something that could affect health. In a clinical research study, the experimental group is exposed to a particular drug or treatment. The control group is not. The number of events in each group is compared to determine relative risk.

Reporting bias

A bias caused by only a subset of all the relevant data being available. The publication of research can depend on the nature and direction of the study results. Studies in which an intervention is not found to be effective are sometimes not published. Because of this, systematic reviews that fail to include unpublished studies may overestimate the true effect of an intervention. In addition, a published report might present a biased set of results (e.g., only outcomes or subgroups where a statistically significant difference was found).

Risk

A way of expressing the chance that something will happen. It is a measure of the association between exposure to something and what happens (the outcome). Risk is the same as probability, but it usually is used to describe the probability of an adverse event. It is the rate of events (such as breast cancer) in the total population of people who could have the event (such as women of a certain age).

Robustness score

A score developed to indicate the number of intervention components hypothesized to be associated with greater treatment effects.

Sensitivity

The ability of a test to identify correctly people with a condition. A test with high sensitivity will nearly always be positive for people who have the condition (the test has a low rate of false-negative results). Sensitivity is also known as the true-positive rate.

Shared medical appointment (SMA)

A group visit where multiple patients are seen together for followup or routine care.

Spearman's correlation

A rank correlation coefficient that is usually calculated on occasions when it is not convenient, economical, or even possible to give actual values to variables but only to assign a rank order to instances of each variable. It may also be a better indicator that a relationship exists between two variables when the relationship is nonlinear.

Specificity

The ability of a test to identify correctly people without a condition. A test with high specificity will rarely be wrong about who *does not* have the condition (the test has a low rate of false-positive results). Specificity is also known as the true-negative rate.

Stages-of-change model

A common health behavioral model consisting of these components: precontemplation, contemplation, preparation, action, and maintenance.

Standard error

The standard deviation of the sampling distribution of a statistic. Measurements taken from a sample of the population will vary from sample to sample. The standard error is a measure of the variation in the sample statistic over all possible samples of the same size. The standard error decreases as the sample size increases.

Standardized mean difference (SMD)

The difference between two estimated means divided by an estimate of the standard deviation. It is used to combine results from studies using different ways of measuring the same concept, e.g. mental health. By expressing the effects as a standardized value, the results can be combined since they have no units.

Statistical significance

A mathematical technique to measure whether the results of a study are likely to be true. Statistical significance is calculated as the probability that an effect observed in a research study is occurring because of chance. Statistical significance is usually expressed as a P-value. The smaller the P-value, the less likely it is that the results are due to chance (and more likely that the results are true). Researchers generally believe the results are probably true if the statistical significance is a P-value less than 0.05 ($p<.05$).

Strength of evidence (SOE)

A measure of how confident reviewers are about decisions that may be made based on a body of evidence. SOE is evaluated using one of four grades: (1) *High* confidence that the evidence reflects the true effect; further research is very unlikely to change reviewer confidence in the estimate of effect; (2) *moderate* confidence that the evidence reflects the true effect; further research may change the confidence in the estimate of effect and may change the estimate; (3) *low* confidence that the evidence reflects the true effect; further research is likely to change the confidence in the estimate of effect and is likely to change the estimate; and (4) *insufficient*; the evidence either is unavailable or does not permit a conclusion.

Summary receiver operating characteristic (SROC)

A data analysis approach that combines independent studies of diagnostic tests. The SROC curve and the area under the curve (AUC) have been proposed as a way to assess diagnostic data in the context of a meta-analysis.

Systematic review

A summary of the clinical literature. A systematic review is a critical assessment and evaluation of all research studies that address a particular clinical issue. The researchers use an organized method of locating, assembling, and evaluating a body of literature on a particular topic using a set of specific criteria. A systematic review typically includes a description of the findings of the collection of research studies. The systematic review may also include a quantitative pooling of data, called a meta-analysis.

Time-series study

A quasi-experimental research design in which periodic measurements are made on a defined group of individuals both before and after implementation of an intervention. Time series studies are often conducted for the purpose of determining the intervention or treatment effect.